# INNOVATIONS IN HEALTH CARE
# FOR PEOPLE WITH INTELLECTUAL
# DISABILITIES

*Edited by*

# Michael Kerr

*Lisieux Hall Publications*

# Other Publications available from Lisieux Hall
(All titles £9.00 + £1.50 p&p)

**Innovations in Evaluating Services for People with Intellectual Disabilities** edited by Roy McConkey.
*The international authorship make this one of the most comprehensive and up-to-date reviews on current thinking about service evaluation. Essential reading for planners and managers.*

**Innovations in Developing Countries for People with Disabilities,** edited by Brian O'Toole and Roy McConkey.
*This important collection of essays ... will provide CBR planners and workers with insight into the rich diversity of CBR initiatives and the importance of leadership and activism by disabled people.* Health Rights

**Innovations in Family Support for People with Learning Disabilities,** edited by Peter and Helle Mittler.
*This book is a must for all professionals working in the field. It will become a key reference volume in the area of family studies.* Frontline

**Innovations in Educating Communities about Learning Disabilities,** edited by Roy McConkey.
*Two features distinguish this addition to the campaigning literature; the selection of often telling cartoons and the emphasis on supporting people with disability labels to be their own ambassadors.* Care Weekly

**Innovations in Educating Children with Severe Learning Disabilities,** edited by John Harris.
*It is rare to read a book about the national curriculum and children with severe learning disabilities that is readable and practical. But this is one such book.* Care Weekly

**Innovations in Employment Training and Work for People with Learning Difficulties,** edited by Roy McConkey & Patrick McGinley.
*Useful practical guide to a number of innovative programmes in vocational training and employment in the UK and other countries.*
Mental Handicap Research

**Innovations in Leisure and Recreation for People with a Mental Handicap,** edited by Roy McConkey & Patrick McGinley.
*Practical and enthusiastic .. can be highly recommended not only to practitioners in the field but to all those wishing to become involved in leisure activities.* International Journal of Rehabilitation Research

# INNOVATIONS IN HEALTH CARE FOR PEOPLE WITH INTELLECTUAL DISABILITIES

**Scarborough Health Authority**

**Library and Information Service**

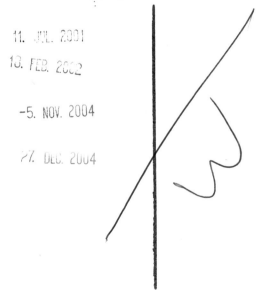

**Innovations In Health Care for People
with Intellectual Disabilities**

**Published by:**

    Lisieux Hall Publications, Whittle-le-Woods, Chorley,
    Lancashire, England, PR6 7DX

Copyright © Lisieux Hall Publications, 1998

Technical Editor: Roy McConkey

A catalogue entry for this book is available from the British
Library.

ISBN 1-870335-23-6

Cover Photo by kind permission of Badaguish: Cairngorm
Outdoor Centre, Aviemore, Scotland.

# INNOVATIONS IN HEALTH CARE
# FOR PEOPLE WITH INTELLECTUAL DISABILITIES

## *Contents*

## SECTION 2: ADVANCES IN MEDICAL SCIENCE

# 1

# *Achieving Health Gain for People with Intellectual Disabilities*

## Michael Kerr

*"Empathy, compassion and action must be the course which the doctor takes. A kind word can make all the difference and alter the course of another person's life."* (a parent)

This quote from a parent of an adult with a learning disability defines three aspects of quality health care for people with a learning disability: (1) attitude, (2) communication and (3) intervention. It also identifies how good quality care will have effects beyond the individual patient. The health, and ill-health, of an individual effects both that individual and the lives of those close to him/her, especially other family members (Todd & Shearn 1996).

Defining the effects of ill-health can be difficult. One way of understanding the potential effect of health (or its absence) on an individual with learning disability and his/her family is to assess the impact of health issues on their quality of life. There is some broad agreement that the basic components of a good quality of life for a person with a learning disability are a combination of certain aspects, or dimensions, of one's life (Blunden 1988; Felce & Perry 1995 ). Four dimensions are commonly emphasised: (1) physical health, (2) social well-being, (3) material well-being and (4) emotional well-being. It is not difficult to see therefore how the effects of a specific illness, such as epilepsy, can influence all these areas; namely causing physical trauma through seizures, restricting socialization, damaging employment opportunities for the individual and the family and through this effecting emotional well-being.

In addition to these dimensions, quality of life is influenced by other factors, in particular an individuals experience and expectations. An individual or family who has tolerated chronic poor health may have little expectation of recovery and not actively seek it.

Health care for people with a learning disability is a balance between achieving the best possible health and reducing the handicaps that ill health, and in some cases it's treatment, can impose on an individual. Achieving this balance involves the ability to assess and understand a person's needs, while delivering care to an individual that is appropriate to these needs and to treat them as effectively as possible.

This book will look at how advances in these three areas: health care delivery, interventions and assessment for people with a learning disability are helping us to meet these needs. The authors represent a selection of the broad range of professionals involved in the delivery of health care to people with a learning disability; coming as they do from the fields of medicine, dentistry, nursing, education and psychology.

Of course, health care does not exist in a vacuum. Both families and professionals delivering care to an individual are effected by broader issues in health care. It is, therefore, necessary to set the scene for care delivery. I will discuss here how the issues of: philosophy of care, health policy, health targets, clinical effectiveness and the role of primary care are influencing and driving the care agenda.

## *Philosophical barriers?*

A person with a learning disability has the same right to a good quality of health as any other individual. This is not to be confused with saying that both require the *same* health care, a so called 'ordinary service'. For health care should be applied individually and related to the needs of that individual.

Unfortunately any discussion on health care relating to people with a learning disability, or its delivery, can easily be overtaken by fears over what is seen as an unacceptable application of the medical model, and thus a reinforcing of stigmatization and a barrier to ordinary lives. Whether or not such fears are justified there can be no doubt that their existence can hinder the advancement of health care for people with a learning disability. More importantly they can serve to camouflage the real barriers to health provision: knowledge, economic priorities, communication and difficulties in the delivery of health care.

As professionals we need to be aware of these philosophical trends, apply them practically and, importantly, heed the words of the parent quoted above; namely understand the constructive power of good communication and empathy, and the creation of a positive attitude.

## Health Gain and Health Care Policy

Three major drives in national health policy will increasingly shape our delivery of health care to people with a learning disability. These are, firstly, the move towards accountability and prioritization through setting *targets*. Secondly, the move towards a health care system built up on proof of interventions, the *clinical effectiveness* movement. Lastly the shift of health care delivery from hospital based secondary care facilities to primary health care teams: a *primary care led* health service. Some understanding of these issues and how they relate to people with a learning disability is needed in order to see the context for endeavouring to improve and maintain the health of this group of individuals.

### Targets

The setting of health targets for services serves two main purposes, firstly, it prioritizes certain health interventions as being more worthy than others and, secondly, it sets an expectation that measurement will occur so that information is available as to whether the target has been met. In all the examples of target setting to date it has been the prioritization of issues which has driven change because measurement has not been actively supported.

Two key documents in the United Kingdom on health delivery for people with a learning disability have advocated a target driven approach; the *Protocol for Investment in Health Gain: Mental Handicap (Learning Disabilities)*, (Welsh Office 1992) and the *Health of the Nation: a strategy for people with learning disabilities* (Department of Health 1995).

The *protocol* focuses on a Health Gain approach. Under the auspices of the Welsh Health Planning Forum, individuals with a learning disability, advocates, representative groups and health professionals advised on necessary targets. These follow a structure with three main features. *Health Gain focused*, improving both the quality and the longevity of life. *People centered*, valuing people as individuals. *Resource effective*, achieving a cost effective balance in the use of available resources.

Health gain targets reflect areas where current opinion, supported by evidence, recognizes both an increased need and that effective interventions exist to address this need. In addition to health gain targets, service targets exist to identify possible service modifications to achieve health gain.

In contrast to the *Welsh Protocol* the *Health of the Nation strategy* highlights areas of importance and possible methods to achieving these, such as health surveillance, but does not set precise numerical targets.

Within the United Kingdom the content of these two documents will drive the resurrecting of services. Key point box one summarizes target setting for people with learning disability.

## Key Points 1: Targets

**Two important documents:**

* *Protocol for investment in Health Gain: Mental Handicap*

*(Learning disabilities).*

* *The Health of the Nation: a strategy for people with learning disabilities*

**Targets set by professional and representative groups**

**Targets restricted to measurable outcomes**

**Targets set priorities for health care.**

**Major areas covered by targets are:**
* Health surveillance: Health promotion and screening, e.g. regular health checks.

* Specific health needs: e.g. reduction in challenging behavior, assessing sensory problems, reducing the side effects of antipsychotic drugs.

* Service delivery: Key workers, transition to adult care.

**Targets will need to be reviewed**

**Targets should be evidence based**

### Clinical Effectiveness

The Clinical effectiveness approach, also known as the Cochrane Collaboration (Welsh Office, 1996), focuses on two issues, firstly an aim that all interventions used by medical practitioners should be proven to work and, secondly, that this evidence, when available should mean that the intervention is implemented into practice. Not unreasonable aims one would feel. In fact, the drive to clinical effectiveness and the closely allied evidence-based medicine, both complement target setting; for example the Welsh Health Gain Targets are evidence based.

The quality of the evidence should be based on both the methodology used and the outcomes measured. Few high quality trials have been performed into the health care of people with a learning disability. So often the impact of our interventions has to be inferred from trials in people without learning disability; presuming they exist. As carers and practitioners we will increasingly needing to assess the interventions we are using. Key point two summarises the main factors in assessing evidence.

## Key Points 2:
### Assessing treatments : A hierarchy of evidence

**Features of good evidence**:
- Chosen from a good sample; representative of the population
- Use of control populations,
- Studies are prospective or cover a long period of time,
- Treatments are randomised to avoid bias,
- They use outcomes relevant to people with a learning disability.

**Features of poor evidence:**
- No control procedures used,
- They report personal opinion not the results of trials,
- Outcomes are ill defined,
- no randomization,
- no measures are taken to avoid bias.

### Primary care

The move to a primary care led health service is not unique to the United Kingdom and is occurring worldwide at varying rates. Its relevance to the healthcare of people with a learning disability has of course been heightened as it is occurring in tandem with deinstitutionalisation. The chapter by Hayward in this book will address the issue in more detail.

It is important to note that the general practitioner, and primary health care team, will be the focus for health delivery to people with learning disability and hence an ability to work within, and a knowledge of, the primary care system will be essential for any professional working with people with a learning disability.

A central feature of a health service led by primary care is the concept of locality purchasing which in turn links up with the target setting noted above. Local areas will set their own targets and standards for health care and buy health care appropriately. This shift of power from central boards has led some to voice concern that the needs of people with learning disabilities would be overlooked, especially by GPs who act as 'fund-holders' (Russell & Paton 1995). Fortunately such fears have not been realized and there is little to suggest that the majority of primary health care teams aim to discriminate in any way against the learning disabled.

This is not to say that the move towards a primary care led health service does not present challenges (see Key point box three). Of particular concern is the gap between the evidence which suggests that active health promotion is essential through some sort of regular screening and the current scientific evidence which suggests that primary care is not delivering, nor expecting to deliver such care (see Hayward in this volume; Kerr *et al* 1996a). We must hope that the drive for clinical effectiveness will influence this current lack of application of evidence.

## Key Points 3:
## Responding to a Primary Care-led Health System

**Positive aspects:**
- Local services for local needs
- Locality purchasing: the community sets its own agenda and standards
- Less stigma?

**Negative aspects**
- Currently not delivering expected health care
- Will need close links to meet specialist need
- Will need proactive health checking, this will need funding
- 'On-demand' system not suited to people with poor communication
- Competing in setting priorities

## *Delivering Health Care - Whose Responsibility?*

In the British Health service the responsibility for accessing health care is the individual's in the majority of circumstances. Thus we have an on-demand health care system. There are of course exceptions where general practitioners, and others, recall individuals for various screening procedures such as child surveillance, immunizations, well women/man clinics and screening for the over 75s. At first sight such an on-demand system does not meet the needs of people with a learning disability as problems with communication and mobility would seem to reduce the ability for individuals to be their own health advocates. The available evidence appears to back up a poor level of both health promotion and untreated illness in people with a learning disability (see Kerr *et al* 1996b for a review). This is despite at least average attendance at surgery as compared to the general population.

How can this be resolved? A starting point is to find out why it occurs. It would appear that a range of factors are playing a role in perpetuating this situation. Firstly, as discussed by Butler in her chapter, individuals with a learning disability, and often their carers, are poor advocates for their health. Active measures are needed to ensure that the importance of health care is explained to individuals with a learning disability. The role of carers - both family and professionals - as front line advocates for health also needs clarifying.

Secondly, health professionals need to understand how the system is failing. We are poor at allowing patients to access our care, we are poor at communicating issues to them and their families and we are poor at talking to each other. We need to develop and deliver appropriate treatments. As the parent said in the opening quotation of this chapter, people want *outcomes* and research into delivering outcomes is needed. In particular, health needs must be prioritised by those who finance care; in particular clinical effectiveness will need funding and primary health care teams will need to be resourced if health surveillance is to become a reality.

## Conclusion

Health care is forever changing, the speed of advancement of knowledge is too much for most professionals. This book will, I hope, serve as a tool for delivering some of these advancements and therefore help in putting them into practice. Advances in the new genetics, brain imaging and assessment of the relationship between brain and behavior are dramatically changing our assessment of individuals with learning disability. Real advancements in treatments are adding to health gain in areas such as epilepsy, psychiatric ill health and sleep disturbance. The application of this knowledge through our primary care systems is a challenge which must be taken on, and funded, by support and professional services. Improvements in health education will allow for this to be explained and for the individuals to have informed choice. Through these innovations health gain for people with a learning disability will begin to occur.

## References

Blunden, R. (1988). Pragmatic features of quality services. In M.P. Janicki, M.W. Krauss & M.M. Seltzer (eds) *Community Residences for Persons with Developmental Disabilities: Here to Stay.* Baltimore: Paul H. Brookes.

Department of Health (1995). *The Health of the Nation: A Strategy for People with Learning Disabilities.* HMSO: Oldham.

Felce, D. & Perry, J.(1995). Quality of life: Its definition and measurement. *Research in Developmental Disabilities.* 16, 51-74.

Kerr. M. Dunstan, F. & Thapar, A. (1996a). Attitudes of general practitioners to caring for people with learning disability. *British Journal of General Practice,* 46, 92-94.

Kerr, M., Fraser, W. & Felce, D. (1996b). Primary health care for people with a learning disability. *British Journal of Learning Disabilities,* 24, 2-8.

Russell, T. & Paton, N. (1995). Are you too expensive for your GP? *Disability Now,* January 1995.

Todd, S. & Shearn, J. (1996). Struggles with time: the careers of parents with adult sons and daughters with learning disabilities. *Disability & Society,* 11, 379-401.

Welsh Health Planning Forum (1992). *Protocol for Investment in Health Gain: Mental Handicap (Learning disabilities).* Cardiff: Welsh Office NHS.

Welsh Office (1996). *Clinical Effectiveness Initiative in Wales: Briefing Paper 2.* Cardiff, Welsh Office NHS.

**Michael Kerr** is Senior Lecturer in Neuropsychiatry at the Welsh Centre for Learning Disability. Dr. Kerr trained both as a general practitioner and as a psychiatrist. He works in epilepsy care, neuropsychiatry and the health care of people with a learning disability.

**Contact Address**
Welsh Centre for Learning Disabilities
Meridian Court
North Road
Cardiff CF4 3BL
Wales, U.K.

# 2

# *Accessing Primary Health Care:*
# *Pathways To Care*

## Brandon Hayward and Michael Kerr

The aim of this chapter is to consider the health needs of people with intellectual disabilities and it will focus on the 'why' and 'how' an individual may access primary health care. We will also address the ways in which all parties including individuals, families, health professionals, and paid and unpaid carers can work cooperatively to improve both the level of health uptake and the quality of service provided. The main theme will be about providing practical supports to general practitioners in the delivery of primary health care to people with intellectual disabilities rather than advocating radical changes to the current practices in primary healthcare systems.

The general practitioner is the professional most often contacted by people with intellectual disabilities and their families or carers (Evans et al 1994) and has always been the major provider of health care to this group. An average practice of 7,500 population will have approximately 150 individuals with intellectual disability, and 30 with severe intellectual disability on their list given prevalence rates of 2% and 0.4% respectively. Such a practice is likely to have 4 general practitioners each seeing approximately 7 - 8 individuals with severe intellectual disabilities. It is clear therefore that the average general practitioner will have little experience of working with people with significant intellectual disabilities and may be forgiven for not viewing this relatively small group as a priority.

The way in which people with intellectual disability access quality health care is becoming increasingly relevant as social policy imperatives lead to the decommissioning of the long stay hospitals and people with intellectual disabilities take their place in the community in ever increasing numbers. For example, in the period 1971 - 1991 the population of hospitals for people with intellectual disability has halved to 30,000 (Mental Health Foundation, 1993).

Given the recent shift towards a primary care led N.H.S. the attitudes of general practitioners to providing care to individuals with intellectual disability are increasingly important. Kerr, Dunstan & Thapar (1996) surveyed attitudes of general practitioners in Wales and found that they accepted that they are responsible for the medical care of people with intellectual disabilities in the community. They did not feel that patients with intellectual disabilities produced greater demand on their time at present, but that the impetus of increased community presence through the resettlement from long stay hospitals would definitely impact on their time. Despite poor communication skills and cognitive deficits, individuals with intellectual disabilities have the same consultation times as others in the community. This may be due to their ignorance about available services (i.e. not knowing what to ask for), and/or a lack of advocacy to question the general practitioner about areas of diagnosis, treatment, and impact on lifestyle of their condition.

## The Need to Access Primary Health Care

People with intellectual disabilities have the same illnesses as everyone else but also have problems with communication and may need additional supports to achieve good health and remain healthy. The access to primary care is a reactive process (Wilson & Haire 1990), i.e. an individual needs to recognise the symptoms of ill-health and be able to seek help and comply with treatment. This model is significantly affected when an individual experiences problems of communication and understanding. Impaired communication which is associated with intellectual disability to varying degrees impacts on the health status of this population, resulting in the under-reporting of physical and mental symptoms (Kinnell 1987).

Often behaviours replace language as the main communication tool of people with severe intellectual disabilities and maladaptive behaviours may be the individual's means of communicating the symptoms of illness. Anxiety about seeing a doctor may manifest behaviourally which can compromise the consultation process and disrupt the surgery environment, Howells (1986) identified that 10% could not be managed in the surgery setting. The manner in which individuals, especially the more severely disabled, are accommodated within the system will have a significant impact on the subsequent level of uptake of health care. General practitioners, and the team including receptionists should be aware of the issues of interaction with people with intellectual disability. Poor or inappropriate communication and a lack of confidence in these situations may well be viewed as being either uncaring or patronising by individuals, families and carers.

Although people with intellectual disabilities have a similar range of morbidity as the remainder of the population, some conditions are seen more frequently in this group. In some cases these conditions are associated with specific syndromes the remainder being a more general distribution within this population.

### Morbidity Associated With Specific Syndromes

Down Syndrome best illustrates this point where there exists a heightened susceptibility to infectious diseases and significantly higher incidence of a number of conditions including - cardiovascular disease, respiratory disease, ocular disorders, leukaemia, hypothyroidism, dental, oral and peri-oral problems and Alzheimer's disease (Lott & McCoy, 1992). People with Down syndrome experience twice the rate of dementia as the general populace (Lund 1985) with earlier onset.

Fragile X is the most common inherited cause of intellectual disability; accounting for 10% of the population group (Webb et al 1986), and epilepsy occurs in approximately 20% of these individuals (Turk et al 1994). Other conditions associated with Fragile X include cardiac abnormalities and joint hyper-extendability (Kerr, Frazer & Felce 1996), and there are also deficits in communication (Hirst et al 1992).

### Morbidity In The Intellectually Disabled

Epilepsy is the most serious neurological condition with a prevalence rate of 0.5 - 0.75% in the general population (Oxley & Smith, 1991). The association with intellectual disability is approximately 33% and 40 - 50% in the more severely disabled, and is particularly prevalent in : Tuberous Sclerosis where it is greater than 90% (Gomez, 1979), Down Syndrome with a 10% prevalence (Collacott, 1993), and Autism with a 30% prevalence (Gillberg & Steffenberg, 1987). As hospital populations decline and more severely and profoundly disabled individuals live in the community, services will need to respond appropriately. The current and future management of this complex disorder, which has poor levels of treatment outcome in the intellectually disabled, has two significant elements: first, the general practitioner managing the care of those individuals who have either an acceptable level of seizure control or those he is confident to manage, and second, a shared care regime between the general practitioner and specialist services. It may prove expedient to develop specialist epilepsy liaison nurse posts to facilitate the communication process in a shared care environment.

There are other physical disorders with a higher prevalence in people with intellectual disabilities including : obesity and heart disease (Turner & Moss, 1996), hypertension and musculo-skeletal problems (Howells 1986, Beange 1995).

People with intellectual disabilities are vulnerable to mental health problems and psychiatric illness. Mansell (1993) indicates that up to 50% of adults with intellectual disabilities have mental health needs (compared with 25% of the general population). Psychotic conditions constitute approximately 10% of this group.

## Accessing Primary Health Care

The intellectually disabled population is comprised of individuals with a diverse range of skills and competencies that fall within an I.Q. range of 0-19 (Profound) to 70-85 (Borderline). It is essential that this population is not viewed as a homogeneous group but as individuals who differ as much from one another as any other group (Howells & Barker, 1990). This is a problem when devising strategies and protocols for delivering services to specific groups.

Evidence from studies into the health care of people with intellectual disabilities (usually undertaken in training centres) indicate a low level of uptake, paradoxically a situation exists where people with intellectual disabilities experience a higher rate of ill health but have less access to service than the general population. Howells & Barker (1986) found that some disorders were inadequately managed including sensory impairments, epilepsy, obesity, hypertension, and bronchitis. Another study by Wilson and Haire (1990) indicated undiagnosed sensory deficits, and that 50% of the study group suffered unmanaged medical problems.

Proactive health measures and health promotion for people with intellectual disabilities are given a low priority within primary care (Langan et al 1993). Individuals are less likely to receive cervical screening, blood pressure monitoring, and regular immunisation.

A study by Whitfield, Langan and Russell (1996) confirmed this phenomenon and also found that individuals with intellectual disabilities consulted significantly higher for diseases of the central nervous system and of the skin than the control group.

There is evidence of high rates of obesity in this group which combined with increased levels of inactivity and under-engagement suggests that an investment in health promotion measures including advice about healthy lifestyles would be useful and ultimately prove cost effective.

### The Role Of Carers

Those individuals who are more severely impaired are reliant on the skill and knowledge of others including parents, families and carers to intervene on their behalf to access health services when they are unable to identify or communicate symptoms of illness. Their awareness of, and attitude towards all aspects of health including the areas of sexuality and relationships will impact on the level of service uptake and ultimately the quality of life of the individual. All carers both formal and informal must develop self awareness in terms of personal ideology, values and prejudice to ensure the well-being of those in their care. On occasion the principles of Normalisation and Social Role Valorisation and other values based philosophies are misinterpreted and individuals may be denied access to appropriate specialist health services in the quest for " normal " patterns of living. It is essential that social care providers are diligent in the establishment of appropriate training and education of care staff in these complex concepts, it is not acceptable that an individual's well-being is jeopardised because it was " their choice " not to visit the G.P. in a simplistic interpretation of the theory.

There are some basic observations that care providers can undertake that will have a positive impact and complement primary health care including : monitoring the weight of the individual, observing any changes to the menstrual cycle, checking for evidence of ear wax, encouraging effective teeth cleaning routines and where appropriate ensuring spectacles are clean and hearing aid batteries are functional.

Farmer et al (1991) evidenced that 54% of those with severe intellectual disability (approximately 108,000 people) live at home, including 90% of children under 15 years and 40% of adults. This huge burden of care will inevitably impact on the health status of parents and primary care providers need to be aware of this situation.

## *Primary Care- The Way Forward ?*

The provision of health care to individuals with intellectual disabilities is increasingly the remit of primary care teams. It has been evidenced that this group have high levels of hidden morbidity, low levels of health promotion and low rates of consultation allied to significant deficits in communication and understanding.

## Health Screening

Regular medical surveillance provided by general practitioners via contractual obligation, is the vehicle used to address the health needs of other vulnerable groups i.e. those individuals under 5 years and over 75 years and it would appear to be needed for people who are intellectually disabled. There are several formal recommendations for proactive health screening for people with intellectual disabilities including : the Welsh Health Planning Forum (1992), a working party of the Royal College of General Practitioners (R.C.G.P., 1990) and most recently the Mental Health Foundation's report; " Building Expectations ", (1996).

The aims of health surveillance are to identify previously undiagnosed illness (to provide appropriate intervention) and to enhance health promotion. The organisation of surveillance is dependent on the establishing of a practice based register of individuals with intellectual disabilities. A comprehensive register may be developed by searching consultation records over a given period, the use of existing information and liaison with social services who have an obligation to organize registers of people with intellectual disabilities.

The second stage of the process of health surveillance is deciding between opportunistic or organised health care as the method of delivery. It would appear that opportunism may fail given that it would be reliant on individuals actively seeking consultation - a process that is currently unsuccessful in providing good quality health care to people with intellectual disabilities. A research study undertaken by Jones & Kerr (1996) has indicated that the introduction of opportunistic health screening has been of little benefit. Therefore the establishment of organised health care would be the preferred option.

Within the context of organised health care there are three developmental options. Firstly the practice could ensure that all individuals with intellectual disabilities on their register were invited to participate in the health promotion initiatives already existing within the framework of services provided by the practice e.g. blood pressure monitoring, well man/woman clinics etc. Secondly a health checking system could be developed without a physical examination and thirdly health checking including a physical examination.

The option of increased access to already existing health promotion strategies although a laudable and worthwhile venture, would not necessarily identify elements of ill health either physical or mental, including behavioural disturbance.

Health checking without a physical examination would usually comprise a checklist that could be completed annually and retained in the patient's notes to identify any changes in their health status. This initiative may find more favour with general practitioners as it would not be very time consuming, although its validity could be questioned without a physical examination.

The third option of a comprehensive health check including a physical examination would be the desirable tool for enhancing the health profile of people with intellectual disabilities by quality health surveillance. The administration of the health check would take approximately 30-40 minutes of the general practitioner's time which could prove extremely cost effective in terms of working proactively and identifying potential problems at an early stage.

### Healthy Alliances

The model of integrated health and social care is fundamental to the provision of quality health care, comprehensive health surveillance should include aspects of social care provision. Social services departments are major sources of referral to primary health care through residential, day services and keyworkers/case managers, and it is essential that healthy alliances exist between agencies, and that they work in partnership to maximise the potential for health gain for people with intellectual disabilities. Health professionals working in multi agency support teams can be utilised to help manage the interface between the services and enhance communication. The primary health care teams should be viewed as significant members of those support teams.

A comprehensive health check could be integrated within the holistic assessment processes of case management or other planning initiatives. The Cardiff Health Check Project is a three year project currently approaching its termination that is jointly undertaken by The University of Wales Department of Psychological Medicine, The Mental Handicap in Wales Applied Research Unit and South Glamorgan (now Cardiff and the Vale of Glamorgan) Social Services. This project has endeavoured to establish whether annual health checks performed by volunteer general practitioners across South Glamorgan will improve health care for people with intellectual disabilities.

Subjects have received three health checks (active group) or two (controls), and the programme has been linked to the individual planning process. Keyworkers have facilitated the process, from recruiting individuals to participate in the project to organising the appointments and accompanying them to the health check and supporting them through its entirety. A total of 56 individuals have received health checks of whom 38 were organised by community nurses and a further 9 were indirectly established by community nurses, confirming the significance of this specialist nursing provision to the delivery of quality health services to people with intellectual disabilities.

Those individuals who have been in receipt of the health checks have been a representative group of varying levels of ability within the intellectual disability range, from mild to profound impairment. None have left the study and the preliminary feedback from individuals has shown that they have an interest in being healthy and viewed the screening process favourably (apart from some insensitive comments from a minority of general practitioners).

### Planning For Acute Morbidity

Central to the process for planning for acute morbidity in the intellectually disabled population is the relationship between the primary health care team, carers, specialist clinicians and the community support teams. A proactive approach to health need is essential, with the general practitioner in the central role. The general practitioner needs to have a knowledge of the predictable morbidity for example those individuals with poorly controlled epilepsy who may require intervention for cluster seizures or status epilepticus. Then often in consultation with specialist clinicians they are able to construct management plans for intervention that may prevent hospital admission.

An integrated, seamless service is paramount to achieving optimum levels of health for people with intellectual disabilities, and carers need to have the health status of the individual as a priority in whatever " life planning " system that is used. Families and carers may need training and ongoing support in the observation of manifestations of illness that are relevant to the individual.

## *The Resettlement Process And Primary Care*

Primary health care teams are expected to meet the health needs of the intellectually disabled in ever increasing numbers as the hospital populations decline in line with resettlement initiatives. These individuals will not become integrated into community based health care systems and receive optimum levels of service without comprehensive support, it is not acceptable to expect primary care teams to merely absorb this challenging group because they now live 'in the community'. Social services and other social care providers, specialist health services and primary health care teams must liaise to ensure an equitable service for people with intellectual disabilities.

In terms of providing health care to individuals resettled from hospital care there are practical methods of facilitating the process that can have a positive impact.

Resettlement managers should be sensitive to the needs of general practitioners and avoid clustering groups around one practice, although housing costs may impact on this decision. A general practitioner who shows a particular interest in this client group should also be given similar consideration if that interest is to be nurtured and developed. Overloading a particular practice will inevitably sour the relationship.

Prior to discharge a health professional from a community team should meet with the general practitioner to discuss the potential referral giving a clear account of the identified health needs of the individual, highlighting the level of support that the individual is likely to receive in the community and negotiating support available for the primary health care team.

On discharge the general practitioner should receive a comprehensive health assessment completed by a hospital clinician. The individual should be supported in the initial contact with the primary health care team by someone with a significant relationship and comprehensive knowledge of the subject. Thereafter the social care providers should be encouraged to view appointments with the general practitioner as a priority and provide the appropriate supports.

Ongoing education and training should be available to care providers in all aspects relating to the health needs of those in their care. They should be well versed in the management of relevant conditions and the use of prescribed medications. Behaviour disturbance for example may be an adverse effect of psychotropic medication, including paradoxical hyperactivity from the use of tranquillisers, and dystonia, tardive dyskinesia, akathisia and akinesia from antipsychotic medication. The provision of this training should be a core functions of community nurses working in specialist community support teams.

A survey of care staff in the west midlands highlighted that challenging behaviour and aspects of safety were the major topics requiring further training (Smith et al., 1996).

## Conclusions

The health needs of people with intellectual disabilities present increasing challenges to primary health care services (Cumella et al 1992), and those individuals may not get an equitable service in terms of consultation and health promotion (Howells 1986, Wilson & Haire 1990, Langan et al 1993).

To respond to this situation the following areas of service development could be considered :

### Training

The Royal College of General Practitioners (1990) advocated undergraduate and post graduate training for primary care practitioners in the management of patients with intellectual disabilities.

This should enhance the communication between the practitioner and the individual, often deficits in communication may exacerbate conditions as individuals are unable to describe symptoms and understand what they should do.

### Improved Communication between Primary Care and Social Services

Multi agency support teams provide ongoing support through holistic assessment to individuals some of whom have complex health needs and multiple disability and also behaviour disturbance and mental illness. They are responsible for coordinating care on a local basis for individuals.

The relationship between these services and primary health care needs to be enhanced. At the very least the general practitioner should have an awareness of the patient's keyworker or point of contact within the team who could provide insights into the level of social care provision etc. If a patient presents as being depressed or withdrawn a conversation with the keyworker could indicate high levels of inactivity and under engagement which could be exacerbating the situation and are quite easily remedied without recourse to treatment.

Specialist clinicians e.g. psychiatrists in intellectual disability, should be sector based covering a defined geographical area with a significant input into community based teams. They have a pivotal role in the provision of health services to the intellectually disabled.

### The Surgery Environment

"G.P.'s should give attention to the atmosphere of their surgery for people with learning disabilities " Mental Health Foundation (1996). Enhanced levels of communication and improved attitudes on the part of all members of the primary care team will have a significant impact on service uptake.

## Information Systems

Comprehensive registers should be developed that are accessible to primary care teams. These registers should include information about others involved in the care of the individual including specialist health services and social care providers.

## Health Checks

Primary health care teams need to establish protocols for inclusive health screening for people with intellectual disabilities, based on contractual obligation. The checks could be facilitated by specialist community nurses and case managers from community support teams.

Without the development of specialist supports and surveillance tools it appears that the reactive processes of primary health care services will inadvertently preclude the intellectually disabled from accessing quality health services.

## *References*

Beange, H., McElduff, A., & Baker, W. (1995). Medical Disorders of Adults with Mental Retardation : A Population Study. *American Journal on Mental Retardation.* 99, 595-604.

Collacott, R.A. ( 993). Epilepsy, Dementia and Adaptive Behaviour in Down's Syndrome. *British Journal of Psychiatry.* 93.

Cumella, S., Corbett, J.A., Clarke, D., & Smith, B. (1992). Primary Healthcare for People with a Learning Disability. *Mental Handicap.* 20, 123-125.

Evans,G., Todd, S., Beyer, S., Felce, D. & Perry, J. (1994). Assessing the impact of the All-Wales Mental Handicap Strategy : A survey of four districts. *Journal of Intellectual Disability Research.* 38, 109-133.

Farmer, R., Rhode, J. & Sachs, B. (1991). *Dimensions of Mental Handicap.* London : Charing Cross and Westminster Medical School.

Gillberg, C., & Steffenberg, S. (1987). Outcome and prognostic factors in Infantile Autism and similar conditions. *Journal of Autism and Developmental Disorders.* 17, 273-287.

Gomez, M. ( Ed.). ( 1979) *Tuberous Sclerosis.* New York : Raven Press.

Hirst, M., Suthers, G., & Davies, K. (1992). X-linked mental retardartion : The Fragile-X Syndrome. *Hospital Update.* 18, 736-742.

Howells, G. (1986). Are the medical needs of mentally handicapped people being met? *Journal of the Royal College of General Practitioners.* 36, 449-453.

Howells, G., & Barker, M. (1990). A protocol for primary health care. *Primary Care for People with a Mental Handicap, occasional paper 47,* 12-13. Royal College of General Practitioners.

Jones, G., & Kerr, M.P. (1996). A randomised controlled trial of opportunistic health screening in Primary Care for people with a Learning Disability-preliminary results. *Abstracts of the 10th World Congress of the International Association for the Scientific Study of Intellectual Disabilities.* ISBN. 951-580-173-177p 264.

Kerr, M.P., Dunstan, F., & Thapar, A. (1996). Attitudes of general practitioners to caring for people with learning disability. *British Journal of General Practice.* 46, 92-94.

Kerr, M.P., Fraser, W.I., & Felce, D. (1996). Primary Health Care for People with a Learning Disability. *British Journal of Learning Disabilities.* 24, vol1, 2-8.

Kinnell, D. (1987). Community medical care of people with mental handicaps. *Mental Handicap.* 15, 146-150.

Langan, J., Russell, O., & Whitfield, M. (1993). *Community Care and the General Practitioner : Primary Health Care for People with Learning Disabilities.* Bristol : Norah Fry Research Centre.

Lott, I. & McCoy,E. (1992). *Down Syndrome : Advances in Medical Care.* New York : Wiley.

Lund, J. (1985). Epilepsy and psychiatric disorder in mentally retarded adults. *Acta Psychiatrica Scandinavica.* 72, 557-562.

Mansell, J.L. (1993). *Services for People with Learning Disabilities, Challenging Behaviour or Mental Health Needs. Project Group Report.*

Oxley, J., & Smith, J. (1991). *The Epilepsy Reference Book.* London : Faber and Faber.

Royal College of General Practitioners. (1990). *Primary care for people with a mental handicap. occasional paper 47.* London : R.C.G.P.

Smith, B., Wai-Ling W., & Cumella, S. (1996). Training for Staff Caring for People with Learning Disability. *British Journal of Learning Disabilities.* 24, 20-25.

The Mental Health Foundation. (1993). *Learning Disabilities The Fundamental Facts.* London : Mental Health Foundation.

The Mental Health Foundation. (1996). *Building Expectations.* London : Mental Health Foundation.

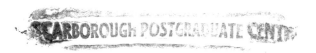

Turk, J. et al. (1994). The Fragile X Syndrome. In Bouras, N. ( Ed.), *Mental Health and Mental Retardation.* Cambrige : Cambridge University Press.

Turner, S., & Moss, S. (1996). The Health Needs of Adults with Learning Disability and The Health of the Nation Strategy. *Journal of Intellectual Disability Research.* 40.

Webb, T., Bundey, S., Thake, A., & Todd, J. (1986). The frequency of the Fragile-X Chromosome among school children in Coventry. *Journal of Medical Genetics.* 23, 396-399.

Welsh Health Planning Forum *(1992) Protocol for Investment in Health Gain : Mental Handicap ( Learning Disabilities ).* Cardiff : Welsh Office NHS Directorate.

Whitfield, M., Langan, J., & Russell,O. (1996). Assessing general practitioner's care of adult patients with learning disability : case-control study. *Quality in Health Care.* 5, 31-35.

Wilson, D., & Haire, A. ( 1990 ). Health care screening for people with mental handicap living in the community. *British Medical Journal.* 301,1379-1380.

**Brandon Hayward** is a clinical nurse specialist working with people who have intellectual disabilities in Cardiff within the context of multi-agency community support teams. His major professional interests lie in the areas of epilepsy, particularly the aspects of treatment outcome and quality of life, and developing coherent systems to facilitate access to primary health care for people with intellectual disabilities.

**Michael Kerr** is Senior Lecturer in Neuropsychiatry at the Welsh Centre for Learning Disability. Dr. Kerr trained both as a general practitioner and as a psychiatrist. He works in epilepsy care, neuropsychiatry and the health care of people with a learning disability.

**Contact Address**
Welsh Centre for Learning Disabilities
Meridian Court
North Road
Cardiff CF4 3BL
Wales, U.K.

# 3

# *Health Care Management and the Individual: Promoting Health*

## Jenny Butler

This chapter on promoting health is divided into two parts. Part one sets the scene for health promotion by describing two specific yet very different health care management programs currently being practiced with people who have intellectual disabilities. These programs, while being successful in themselves, demonstrate problems of overall health education availability.

Part two then questions the ongoing feasibility of such programs and where future directions and developments in promoting health should occur, and offers at least one solution for the future. It is the contention throughout this chapter that as service providers for people with intellectual disabilities it is part of our role to act as 'information sieves' or as the 'middle man' between health promotion, education and the individual.

## 1. HEALTH CARE MANAGEMENT PROGRAMMES

### The Role of Health Care Providers

The main role of health care providers with people who have intellectual disabilities is for them to act as 'information sieves' or as the 'middle-man'. This means being an effective communicator and providing information and education in both informal and formal ways.

The basic rules for effective communication are:

- focus............on the individual,
- assess...........what information the person needs and/or requires,
- modify..........the information to suit individual needs,
- explain.........demonstrate, describe and practise,
- evaluate........ .the success or otherwise of the information-giving
- repeat.......... .if necessary.

The above theory is straight forward and quite self-explanatory. It is the implementation of the rules that is important. In order to best illustrate how these rules can operate, two specific documented health education programs are detailed below.

## Health Education for Cervical Smear Test

Two sisters, both in their late 30s, with mild to moderate intellectual disabilities were taken to the local Family Planning Clinic by their case manager/social worker to be seen for women's health screening ie: cervical smear testing. The doctor was unable to perform the tests as both women were fearful of and unfamiliar with the procedure. They also refused to be parted from each others company. The sisters were referred to the educational counselor for people with intellectual disabilities who worked in the same building.

**Focus**: The multi-disciplinary team consisting of the doctor, the case manager/social worker and the educational counsellor worked in conjunction with the sisters, and the following health education program, in line with their physical and medical needs was developed.

**Assessment:** Individual assessments were initially completed by the counselor to assess the sisters general sexual knowledge. Each assessment included establishing whether or not they had been or were currently sexually active.

The women were both currently sexually active and by their own initiative or that of their partners were practising safe sex. They were found to have a reasonable knowledge of sexuality and sexual health issues, but had little or no understanding of the cervical smear test procedure. Both sisters had a low level of literacy skills which did not allow them to adequately understand generic written literature.

**Modify:** The counselor had previously developed an instructional guide which was both pictorial and written in easy to understand language. This guide together with relevant videos were used to explain the procedure. The content of the sessions included education about positioning for examination, instruments used, what the doctor actually does and why the procedure is so important.

**Explain:** Over the next few weeks educational sessions were conducted in the same clinic room in which the procedure would take place. The sisters were introduced to the doctor, (a woman as they requested), who would perform the tests. A series of instant photos were taken which were added to a pictorial information folder during the weekly sessions. Photos included pictures of the doctor, the two sisters, the room and instruments. This folder was taken home, so that during the following week the case manager/social worker could reinforce what they had learnt during the previous sessions. A step by step demonstration was given by the counselor and these steps were practiced until the sisters were comfortable about what was going to happen during the procedure. After choosing whom they would like as a support person, and having been reassured that they could attend together, an appointment was made with the doctor.

**Evaluate:** The first appointment was to familiarise the sisters with the formality of having the doctor present and was in effect a dress rehearsal. Whilst the educational sessions were being conducted the doctor was kept updated on the progress of these formal strategies.

After seven weeks the cervical smear tests were performed. This method of instruction proved to be successful for both sisters, but a "hiccup" occurred for one of the women when one of the very much rehearsed steps was omitted by the doctor. The doctor had failed to place a sheet across her abdomen. The doctor made amends by following the steps as previously practiced, and from there the test resumed without incident.

The need to **Repeat** was required throughout the instructional and practice stages of the entire program.

## Health Education: Prisoner Health Promotion Project.

At a maximum security prison in a large city in Australia, a unit has been developed for prisoners identified as having an intellectual disability. The unit aims to provide a safe environment for prisoners with an intellectual disability, provide opportunities for them to address offending behaviour, and to develop skills which will enhance the prisoners ability to re-enter the community upon release.

The unit houses up to 22 prisoners with intellectual disabilities, who are mostly in the borderline to moderate range of intellectual disability and who have committed offenses such as murder, rape, child sex offenses, arson, burglaries and other crimes. The unit also houses two non-disabled mainstream prisoners, called 'stabilisers', who provide personal and practical support to prisoners. Mainstream prisoners have to submit a written application and then be interviewed to assess their suitability for the 'stabiliser' position.

**Focus:** The health needs of these prisoners are the same as for any other male. However, being in prison presents health issues which require intervention and education using creativity when working in an environment with such strict rules and policies. The particular health needs pertinent to being accommodated in a large institution include personal hygiene, safe sexual practice, and protection against infectious diseases. A major concern in the prison is the occurrence of sexual activity when prisoners are confined to their cells. Prison policy states that sexual practices are prohibited in the prison and therefore no safety measures, such as distribution of condoms, are provided. Prisoners with an intellectual disability are engaging in sexual activity with little recognition or concern for the risks involved. Prisoners are often directed to change cells, which adds to the risks related to having multiple partners.

**Assessment:** Infection control education is a health program repeated at regular intervals and for new prisoners in this unit. Infection control education covers topics such as strategies to prevent transmission of infectious diseases such as HIV, AIDS, Hepatitis, head lice, tinea, scabies, and other skin diseases. Topics and strategies, taught in detail are safe sex techniques, cleaning syringes and abstinence from sharing needles, early reporting of skin rashes and constant scratching, and listing personal items which are not to be shared (razors, toothbrushes and combs).

**Modify:** The infection control education has been taken from a mainstream education package for the prison population, and modified to suit the learning needs of the prisoner with an intellectual disability. Education is in the form of open discussion and question time. The aim is for prisoners to have increased awareness in the dangers of unsafe sex and drug taking practices. To achieve this aim, the education strategy of peer education has been utilised.

Peer education provides the 'stabilisers' (described above) with the opportunity to increase their own knowledge and skills in leadership and role modeling. The 'stabilisers' are taught information regarding infection control and then shown how to teach this to fellow prisoners. The value of peer education, is that prisoners are being taught by someone they are able to relate to, and in whom they have a feeling of trust.

**Explain:** By using peer education questions can be answered with a level of understanding towards how the prisoner is feeling and the position in which they are in. Peer education is part of the modification used for infection control education in this unit. The unit 'stabiliser' also receives training in communicating with prisoners who have an intellectual disability. The 'stabiliser' is able to articulate the current needs of the prisoners, and then effectively address the issues related to infection control.

One particular issue that has arisen, involved a prisoner, charged with sexual offenses, who has been offering to perform sexual favours for other prisoners. The 'stabiliser' was aware of the situation as the prisoners being offered the favours were informing him of these activities. The 'stabiliser' was then able to pass this information on to the unit's program co-ordinator. The whole unit then received infection control education. The 'stabiliser' delivered the education and encouraged discussion in response to the question "What happens if I have unsafe sex?" Unsafe sex was explained in detail, particularly describing what the prisoner had been offering to fellow prisoners. It was made aware to all prisoners that AIDS can be caught in prison. This seemed to be the only statement that reached the prisoners involved in the sexual activities. A group education session was conducted in order to raise the awareness of all the prisoners, and an individual session to confirm understanding was conducted with the prisoner offering the favours.

**Evaluate:** The effectiveness of the infection control education is difficult to assess, when a great deal of unconfirmed sexual practices still exists in the unit, - even after the education has been delivered. On completion of the program, a formal question sheet was co-actively completed with every prisoner. The questions asked deal with how infectious diseases are transmitted, safe sex practices, strategies to avoid coming in contact with blood, and how to report cases of skin diseases.

The question sheet is divided into two categories. *Category 1* (six questions) relates to questions regarding Infection Control Strategies; *Category 2,* (seven questions) contains questions related to facts regarding HIV, AIDS and Hepatitis.

Out of the 13 prisoners who answered the question sheet for *Category 1,* 4 prisoners had a perfect score, 2 scored five out of the six and 7 scored four out of the six. The average score was 4.8. out of 6.

In *Category 2,* 3 prisoners had a perfect score, 3 scored six out of seven, 3 scored five out of seven, 3 scored four out of seven and 1 scored three out of seven. The average score was 5.3. out of 7.

The results of *Category 1* indicated that the information was presented at a level which developed the prisoner's knowledge and awareness regarding infection control strategies. The prisoners are now aware of strategies to protect themselves from contracting HIV and Hepatitis. However, the area that requires further education is an understanding of which sexual activities are safe.

The results of *Category 2* indicate knowledge of HIV/ AIDS and Hepatitis is also at a very basic level, with prisoners being unaware of **all** the relevant facts related to the diseases. The particular area which continues to cause confusion is in the transmission of HIV/AIDS and Hepatitis. The average score for this category is four, out of a possible seven. This indicates that whilst there has been enough knowledge gained in order to have a basic understanding of infectious diseases, further education would also be of benefit for continuing to increase knowledge and understanding of HIV / AIDS and Hepatitis.

The conclusion of these results recommended that regular sessions of this nature should take place. This would enable the ever changing population in this unit to benefit from knowing this information. Regular sessions would also give those who scored quite low in the quiz, an opportunity to clarify areas of confusion and consolidate what they have learnt. This repeat learning would also be of assistance in the prisoners' retaining information.

**Repeat:** These recommendations were followed, however, unsafe sexual practices continue in the unit and some prisoners admit to unsafe practices when released from prison. The difficulty appears to be in the prisoner's retaining the information and then acting upon it. That is being able to put 'theory into practice'. Health education and promotion to this client group requires repetition and a constant role model, such as the 'stabiliser' and the utilisation of peer education. The unit continues to try to increase the prisoner's awareness of these particular health issues and to increase their acceptance of responsibility for their actions in guarding themselves against infectious diseases.

## *Writing up a Health Promotion Programme*

The rules for effective communication noted at the outset of this chapter offer a formal structure for writing up any health promotion program, e.g. for exercise and diet. The rules themselves offer relevant sub-headings that act as a 'checks and balances' to ensure some degree of achieving what you set out to communicate. Each rule is both necessary and essential, and therefore no rule should be omitted.

Other health promotion programs can be cross checked for "effective communicating" by turning these basic rules into a checklist.

- Is the program addressing individual needs?
- Have you assessed what is needed to be taught ?
- Has the program been modified to suit the abilities of the learner ?

- Are adequate and appropriate instructions, demonstrations and practice written into the program ?
- Is an evaluation method built into the program design ?
- Are opportunities for repeat learning built into the program ?

Informal education opportunities arise at any time, and are often spontaneous and conversational. The best approach here is to be natural and as the name suggests, informal. Pre-planning of such opportunities is (and more often than not) out of the question. However in evaluating your own performance on how such opportunities were handled retrospectively, the rules of thumb again offer a structure to rate effectiveness.

- Did I focus on the individual?
- Did I assess accurately what is needed to be taught ?
- Did I modify the information to suit the abilities of the learner ?
- Were adequate and appropriate instructions, demonstrations and practice offered ?
- Am I able to evaluate what the individual gained / learnt?
- Were opportunities for repeat learning offered ?

## Conclusion

Each of the two practices detailed were in their own way successful. The two women in the first scenario received a great deal of information and had much overdue cervical smear tests performed, which reduced their health risks. They also now have greater confidence in their knowledge and less fear in regard to medical professionals. The experience for both women was very positive and demystifying whereas many other clients and their carers would experience one, or perhaps two, consultations with a professional counselor and be handed pamphlets and brochures to take home and study.

Although the success of the program for prisoners with intellectual disabilities was varied, depending upon the individual, all participants gained some valuable information regarding health risks. For a quarter of the prisoners the program was completely successful, in terms of knowledge acquisition, and for others it demonstrated that a lot more input was needed. It did give facilitators a benchmark from where further explanation and expansion was required.

Both programs owe their degree of success to a multi-disciplinary approach. Staff included doctors, psychologists, social workers and specialist counselors. All these people gave time and expertise to ensure a positive outcome for the participants. Multi disciplinary teams, at their best, are able to provide the following: overall consistency and repetition, opportunities for structured learning in more than one environment, accurate and appropriate health information and a wide range of expertise. They are obviously highly staffed teams of specialists and are generally well resourced. There is no question that this approach is an effective and appropriate way to operate, but it is both time consuming and expensive. This level of involvement is the exception rather than the norm, and the "ideal" option and so a paradoxical situation arises whereby their success is also their limitation.

## 2. FUTURE DEVELOPMENTS

In part one, the two health education programs which were discussed proved to be successful. The first of these programs was the result of a medical referral, and it goes with out saying, that the second program involved a 'captive' audience. The second program was also viewed as a vital component of high profile community problems and an essential part of rehabilitative education. However, both programs were designed to react to existing and acknowledged problems and deficits. They were not in themselves preventative or proactive programs.

People with intellectual disabilities generally experience the same health needs and medical problems as their non-disabled peers. What they do not have is the same access to accurate and reliable information that is appropriate for their level of understanding or abilities. The vast majority of health promotional advertising material is aimed at the 'average' intelligence level of the general population. A population which by and large has easier access to a wider range of community based and specialist services. In part, this lack of health promotional information specifically designed for people with intellectual disabilities, has meant that people with intellectual disabilities have little or no understanding of their specific and or general day to day health needs or they have a very confused notion of what constitutes health.

What needs to happen is for the vast majority of people with an intellectual disability to have 'some' sort of access to 'some' sort of knowledge and information. Most of us are faced at some point in our lives with a myriad of health information that is daunting to say the least - imagine therefore how difficult it is for someone with an intellectual disability to assess this same information. It is important that people with disabilities are not excluded from learning about health because of their level of disability. Future development needs to recognise and concentrate on the enormous gap that exists in information access. Such development is not intended to replace the intensive multi- disciplinary approach but rather to extend the benefits and advantages that information can offer, especially in a preventative sense rather than a reactionary sense.

## Case Studies

Consider the following two case studies.

**Anna:** *is a thirty five year old, young single woman who has a mild intellectual disability. She attended mainstream school as an integration student until year 7. Anna enjoyed school and has the reading level of an average eight year old. She lives in a group home and attends an adult training centre on a full-time basis. She hasn't a boy-friend currently, but has had several in the past. Anna often goes to the doctor whenever she feels unwell, to re-new a prescription for asthma medication, and for other minor ailments. She has never had a cervical smear test. She doesn't have a regular doctor, but has attended the same large medical practice for over eight years, and is known by them all. Apart from asthma since childhood, and all the other usual childhood illnesses, Anna generally has had good health. Her mother and father both died at relatively young ages. Her father died when she was still a young child from a very sudden heart attack. Her mother died three years ago from breast cancer. Her maternal grandmother also died from breast cancer. Anna has no siblings, and only irregular contact with aunts and cousins. She has one or two close friends who also live in group homes.*

**Cecily:** *is a thirty three year old, young single woman who lives alone and has a full-time job. She is tertiary educated and professionally employed. She has a boy-friend six years older than herself, but they do not live together. Cecily keeps good health and only ever goes to the doctor on the odd occasion she may feel unwell, re-new a prescription for the contraceptive pill, and her cervical smear test every two years. She has attended the same doctor for over ten years, and is very happy with her medical care. Apart from appendicitis at the age of ten, and all the other usual childhood illnesses, Cecily has had exceptional health. Her mother and father are both still living and aged 71. Her father is a diabetic and has been for 35 years, her mother has had osteoporosis for the last 9 years. Cecily's two sisters and brother who are all older than herself have had no unusual medical problems. Cecily has a wide circle of friends and colleagues and regular contact with her family.*

If we compare these two women in relation to how they are able to select and use information about health, we find that Cecily has access to a wide range of material and resources, these include television, documentaries, books, computers, resource centres, professional appointments and social conversations. She is able to use these 'tools' whenever she needs to.

On the other hand, Anna, whilst she may have physical access to the same material and resources as Cecily, she is not able to use the information in the same way. For example: television information (documentaries, soap operas and advertisements) often move too quickly and the concepts are too abstract for her to successfully understand, magazines are generally used pictorially and books are generally above her comprehensive reading level. Children's books are often not age or topic appropriate. Her social conversations as a rule are with people who also have intellectual disabilities.

It is not the intention that Anna should be able to access **all** of this material independently, it is an accepted reality that she, like most people with an intellectual disability, may always need assistance of some description. However, to have at hand specifically designed resources that people with intellectual disability can use either independently or with appropriate service providers would mean that someone like Anna would have a far greater chance of learning and retaining knowledge. Money and time would be well spent now in developing the appropriate health related resources. Such an investment would have a much greater 'shelf' life than a 12 weekly session program.

Adapted written material for people with intellectual disabilities is becoming more common in addressing all sorts of issues, including health. This of course is a wonderful support to staff, carers and families as well as those intellectually disabled people with some reading ability.

Other resources that have already proved successful are audio tapes and videos. Such resources can be used over and over again and are an invaluable aid in repetitious learning that does not always involve precious staff time. Most homes, whether they be private or group homes already have cassettes and video recorders. It won't be long before these houses also have the latest computer equipment.

Given the vast range of sophisticated computer software packages designed for the non reading preschooler and early primary years, it must be possible to devise equally clever, interactive age appropriate programs for people with intellectual disabilities. The programs should involve spoken instructions, games and challenges. They can be touch screen for participants for whom the mouse is to difficult to manoeuvre. More sophisticated and currently available computer programs on 'home medicine' already exist for the Cecily's of this world.

The value of this initially high cost development will not only outlive its worth but would also be cost retrievable through marketing the products at affordable, yet cost covering prices. Research and development in this sphere of work may initially take time for benefits to become obvious, but this has been true for all such work in multi media, and is very much dependent upon advertising and making sure availability is known.

## *Conclusion*

There are many different ways that we can communicate health information and deal with the health issues of people who have intellectual disabilities. What is important to remember is that dignity and respect for the individual should always be paramount. Therefore, there will always be a need for field workers to focus on the individual and to some greater or lesser degree be available to provide appropriate assistance.

The quality of health education is undeniably important, however, reaching as many people as possible must lead future development into finding ways and means of improving accessibility. Concentration on the development of adapted and appropriate health promotion materials will go a long way towards addressing the accessibility of information available for people with intellectual disabilities and their carers.

Time, creativity and expertise utilised now will be both time and cost effective for the future and will benefit a wider range of people with intellectual disabilities.

## *References*

Annison, J., Jenkinson, J., Sparrow, W. & Bethune, E. (1996) *Disability: A Guide for Health Professionals,* Melbourne: Thomas Nelson Australia.

Hawe, P., Degeling, D. & Hall, J. (1994) *Evaluating Health Promotion: A Health Worker's Guide,* Sydney: Maclennan and Petty.

Egger, G., Spark, R. & Lawson J. (1994) *Health Promotion Strategies and Methods,* Sydney: Mc Graw-Hill Book Company.

**Jenny Butler** is a teacher and educational counsellor who works in the Developmental Disability Unit at Monash University, Australia. She has extensive experience in service delivery and systems review. She now provides counseling and service consultancy on health, human relations and sexuality issues in people with intellectual disability.

**Contact Address**

Developmental Disability Unit,
Monash University
Melbourne
Australia

# 4

# *Vision and Hearing in People with Intellectual Disabilities*

## Alison M. Kerr

This chapter aims to share the experience of providing systematic assessments of vision and hearing to 600 people in a large institution in the process of discharging its residents to the community.

Many large institutions in Britain were established at the turn of the century to protect disabled people from exploitation and abuse. Although the intention was humane and the outcome satisfactory in some cases, separation from the mainstream of society has allowed standards of health care to drift below acceptable levels.

Our institution was no exception to the general experience and in 1990 a limited review of health needs indicated that although crisis medical care was being provided and general practitioners carried out the regulation annual examinations, few residents had been offered specialist diagnosis or assessment of their neurological or genetic problems nor testing of their vision and hearing Kerr (1994). At this stage there was scepticism about the value of proactive assessments and concern regarding the quality of health care, was curbed by anxiety about the cost. It was therefore necessary to provide further evidence on the prevalence and significance of health problems.

A vision screening programme for two wards was carried out voluntarily by final year students at the Caledonian University (McCulloch, Sludden, McKeown, Kerr 1996). This culminated in a Vision Week at which Professor Mette Warburg from Copenhagen conducted ophthalmic clinics on several wards and delivered the Halliday Lecture on 'Visual Impairment among people with developmental delay' as the centre piece of a 1993 Symposium in the Royal College of Physicians and Surgeons of Glasgow. At the same event our initial health review was presented and contributions on the nutritional and genetic needs of the residents were provided by consultants from other Glasgow hospitals who had been serving the learning disabled population (Kerr 1994).

The group of senior specialists who contributed to the Symposium agreed to form a Working Party on the Medical Needs of Learning Disabled people, thus providing a multidisciplinary advisory body at medical consultant level which has continued to offer advice to the Health Board and Trust. The Working Party has supported the health initiatives.

In January 1995 we received the promise of sufficient funding from the Greater Glasgow Health Board and Community Mental Health Trust to provide vision and hearing assessments for the residents over a four year period. It was agreed that the primary physician for each ward would retain the responsibility for acting on reports. Our request was refused for a clinical psychologist or occupational therapist to be appointed to assist in clinical audit and liaison. However a speech and language therapist, already fully employed by the hospital was invited to liaise with the project to encourage implementation of the specialists' advice.

The box below summarises the steps involved in undertaking a health assessment and the specific actions undertaken in our project, and the box overleaf gives our recommendations for a vision and hearing team.

---

### Steps in Health Assessment I
*(what we did in brackets)*

- Establish the range of identified health problems (for 60 people)

- Choose specific health problems to be assessed (vision & hearing)

- Persuade the physicians and administration of the need to assess.

- Find specialists with the appropriate skills (optometrist & audiologist)

- Agree project duration (4 years for 600 people) & cost per test (£25) .

- Agree format and circulation of reports (in plain English to all carers)

- Ensure that health providers accept responsibility for follow up action

- Encourage therapy departments to allocate time for liaison.

- Agree the place & requirements for testing (quiet room on wards)

- Ensure that key workers attend appointments with residents.

---

---

**Recommended Vision and Hearing Team**

- Physician co-ordinator (paediatrician in our project)
- Secretary (computer skills invaluable)
- Two audiologists
- Two optometrists
- Liaison speech and language therapist
- Liaison occupational therapist **
- Senior clinical psychologist (not appointed) **

** *team members were asked to give one or two sessions weekly to the project*

---

## Methods

We began work in January 1995 as a small team consisting of one doctor, two audiologists, one - later two - optometrists (opticians), a secretary and a liaison speech and language therapist. Each team member allocated half or one day weekly to the project.

All the tests of vision and hearing are planned to take place on the wards with an experienced nurse in attendance. The specialists arrange each visit flexibly to suit themselves and ward routines; visiting first the wards due for early closure. Wards provide a quiet room for the tests.

The project office is furnished with a computer, independent of the hospital recording system and 'Access' relational database software on which to record data and generate cumulative reports for clinical audit. However paper records are kept also.

The physician begins the process by recording, from the medical case notes and nursing care plans, precise statements of family and developmental history and reports from neurologists, geneticists, hearing, vision and nutrition specialists giving name, date and diagnosis. Other stated medical diagnoses and current medications are listed separately.

Staff opinion is requested regarding each person's level of physical and intellectual impairment and whether visual or hearing impairment, feeding difficulty or seizure disorder are present. This 'Health Check' summary provides pre-test information for the optometrists and audiologists and the data is entered on the computer database for clinical audit. A copy is provided for the primary physician with the recommendation that it be copied for the new general practitioner when a resident moves into the community.

The two audiologists visit together using as far as possible the same instruments as when testing able people. If pure tone audiometry is not possible they use ability related distraction and performance tests looking for responses to sounds of known pitch and intensity. We attach great importance to the attendance of the chief carer with the resident in order to encourage co-operation, convey information about the resident to the specialist and to pass on practical advice from the audiologists to the other members of staff.

The optometrists have visited the wards separately although we have come to feel that it is best if they visit together. They have used conventional vision testing equipment as far as the co-operation of the residents allows but have adapted their methods to suit the clientele. Cardiff cards have been used for testing visual acuity.

The audiometricians and optometrists discuss their findings and advice with the ward staff to ensure that the final recommendations will be acceptable.

In addition to traditional reports, the vision and hearing specialists provide reports in 'plain English', technical terms being used when necessary but explained in lay terms for the benefit of the abler residents and for carers who may be members of the family or from another caring profession. Such a report states any diagnosis which has been made, the likely outcome or prognosis, recommended treatment and the time interval after which the examination should be repeated. Each report gives the name, qualifications and contact address for the specialist and the date of the examination.

The vision and hearing reports are photocopied and delivered to each of those for whom they have been written, namely the primary physicians, therapists and social work teams who are currently placing people in the community. We suggest that a photocopy of the plain English vision and hearing reports may be included, unaltered, in the 'life style' log books which are provided for those moving into the community. A copy of each report is also placed in the medical case file which is kept in the ward.

Additional funding has been obtained to purchase a supply of polyvinyl folders 22x15cm in which to present the plain English reports to a pilot group of residents. These personal 'Health Watch' books are intended to remain with each resident after resettlement in the community and the key carer is advised to take the book with the individual when he or she attends future health specialist appointments. In this way we hope to ensure that the relevant health information is at hand at the next appointment.

We advise that specialists who are consulted in future should be routinely invited to record their advice in plain English for their patient and his or her carer, following the style of the vision and hearing reports. Since this is now becoming accepted as good medical practice for the general population we consider it appropriate that those with intellectual disability should enjoy the same advantage, particularly since they are peculiarly dependent on the cater to provide background health information and carers are apt to change in the community, as in many institutions. The style of report is illustrated in Figure 1.

The liaison speech and language therapist visits the wards after the tests have been reported to discuss the reports and encourage and assist the making of arrangements to obtain aids. She advises key workers when adjustments in ward management are found to be desirable .

Data from the vision and hearing reports is entered by the project secretary into a series of databases related to the health check database.

Periodic written audit reports are circulated to the staff giving the findings of the project in its progress through the hospital. Six monthly seminars are arranged addressing health issues with ward staff taking an active part. By sharing information with all the caring professionals and teaching the principles of health care we aim to encourage good practice in the hospital and in the community as relocation of residents and staff is achieved.

The box below summarises further steps in health assessments and the actions taken on our project.

---

**Steps in Health Assessment II**
*(what we did in brackets)*

- Establish free-standing relational database to store the data (Access)

- Preliminary review of medical records (team physician)

- Ward tests offered in agreed order (30 minutes per person)

- Plain English reports delivered to team physician.

- Immediate copies to primary physicians, therapists & carers

- Plain English reports delivered as property of resident (pilot stage)

- Seminars highlight and discuss health issues (6-monthly)

- Information sharing though reports and publications

- Provide argument and prototype for regional health data base.

---

## About your vision

Your eyesight was tested on .....

Your eyes are healthy but not well focussed for distance and we have supplied you with spectacles which will let you make out the numbers on a car at ...... paces

Your eyes are not well focussed for near vision and your spectacles will help you to see near objects better. The figure below shows the size of object which you can see clearly with spectacles.

**A**

Your lenses are hazy due to cataract and your central vision is not good although your side vision is good. You will find it helpful to move close to things you want to see and a bright light will help you to do close work. you will need assistance in traffic and on possibly on stairs. We have supplied you with one pair of spectacles for both near and distant vision and your name is engraved on them. You are advised to request another vision test in one year.

The lens powers are..... with a near addition of.........
Lost or broken spectacles can normally be replaced or repaired without cost
This report is supplied by Mr... (optician) address......... telephone......... Glasgow
This report was supplied to Jean Smith.........date of birth..........address.......

*page 1*

## About your Hearing

Your hearing was tested on

*page 2*

You have severe hearing loss in both ears and it will help if you are spoken to on the left. It will help if the wax is gently removed from your ears by your doctor or clinic nurse. It will also help if you are able to use a hearing aid and this can be arranged through you doctor and ...............clinic

You are advised to request another hearing test in

Severe bilateral hearing loss means 70-90 decibels of hearing loss
This test was carried out by audiologist ............ address............ telephone.....
This report was supplied to Jean Smith.........date of birth..........address.......

## *Results*

At the midpoint of project 'Health Check', summaries have been completed for 450 of the almost 600 residents and vision tests for 200 (January 1996). The population is ageing as every effort is made to keep disabled young people in the community and the mean ages for the residents are 55 years for men and 57 years for women with a range from 26 to 90 years.

Forty per cent of residents cannot walk unsupported, 35 per cent cannot use their hands without physical assistance in simple self care tasks and 62 percent cannot express themselves in sentences.

The health check reviews found that only 8 per cent of records contained a neurologist's report on the condition underlying the intellectual disability. Some form of genetic screening had been offered to 34 per cent however family and early medical histories indicated that a genetic cause was unlikely in only 14 per cent, probable or certain in 36 per cent and possible in a further 50 per cent, so that screening would be appropriate in 86 per cent of residents.

Seizures have been recorded at some time in 45 per cent of residents and in 32 per cent this remained an active problem. Feeding difficulties or other nutritional problems were present in 56 per cent of residents. Virtually all residents had been recorded as having other medical conditions and many of these were for long-standing irritating or painful conditions such as varicose eczema, peptic ulceration and tinea pedis.

At the beginning of the project ward staff thought that hearing and visual impairments might affect about ten percent of residents however as the testing programme progressed, with staff observing the results, the level of awareness increased. About ten percent of residents were unable to co-operate satisfactorily in the test situation. However with a knowledgeable key worker in attendance it was usually possible to reach an estimate of impairment and provide practical advice.

Of those in whom the level of hearing could be tested, 25 per cent had normal hearing and 75 per cent some reduction in hearing. In 34 per cent of the population tested the hearing loss was mild (30-50 decibels' loss) and in 41 per cent it was moderate, severe or profound (decibel loss of 50-70, 70-90 and over 90 respectively). In 12 per cent of the testable group the level of loss was such as to justify a hearing aid although difficulties in understanding might limit its use and lead to modified recommendations. The advice to remove ear wax was frequently given but this was not considered a major contributor to the hearing losses detected.

The preparation of the vision reports has lagged behind the rest of the programme for reasons outwith the hospital. However earlier vision testing initiatives which spearheaded the current project have supplemented information, giving 200 test reports to date. As with hearing tests about 10 per cent have been unable to co-operate. Ninety five per cent of those able to co-operate have shown some degree of visual defect or were considered likely to benefit from correction with spectacles. The optical diagnoses ranged through simple defects amenable to spectacle correction to complex malformations resulting from the original neurological disorder and its complications. Treatable conditions were common and included conditions of the eyelids, infections and glaucoma. In 11 per cent of residents cataracts required surgery.

It was common to find that one individual had both hearing and visual impairments. Table 1 shows the results of vision and hearing tests in a typical group of residents who were consecutively assessed.

## Practical Observations and Local Issues

Although the final clinical audit of the project is still to come there have been obvious benefits to the residents and ward staff. Spectacles, lens implants for cataract, relief from impacted wax and chronic ear infections, and hearing aids have improved health and quality of life for the residents. There has been heightened staff awareness of the importance of vision and hearing for the residents. Nurses have enjoyed being included in the testing situation and noticed improved communication after treatment of deafness and poor vision. The teaching seminars have introduced ideas from other areas of the country and encouraged cross-disciplinary discussion within this area.

The Vision and hearing reports have been well received and found useful, particularly by the therapy and social work departments in planning future accommodation and care in the community. Demand for information outstrips our capacity for provision of health information. Twenty-five pilot 'Health Watch' booklets have been enthusiastically received by carers in the hospital and community with suggestions that use of further symbols would be welcomed by some people who cannot read but are eager to understand the content. The information was not seen as duplicating health information from other sources.

Ward testing has been a great success, indeed in our situation it presented the only realistic way to proceed. Some adaptations of methods and equipment were necessary but have not generally been problematic. In general the vision and hearing specialists have found that they require twice the usual time allotted for an able person in order to test residents adequately.

| Case No | Right Ear | Left Ear | Left Deafness | Right Deafness | Visual Diagnosis |
|---|---|---|---|---|---|
| 1 | wax | wax | mild | mild | spectacle for distance |
| 2 | intact | reddened drum | severe/profound | severe/profound | toxoplasma retinitis |
| 3 | wax | intact | moderate | moderate | strabismus |
| 4 | intact | intact | normal | normal | bilateral cataract |
| 5 | wax | thickened drum | normal | normal | lens implants |
| 6 | wax | wax | mild | moderate | spectacles prescribed |
| 7 | wax | wax | mild | mild | bilateral cataract |
| 8 | infection | infection | severe | severe | myopic astigmatism |
| 9 | wax | wax | mild/moderate | mild/moderate | cataract & keratoconus |
| 10 | wax | wax | inconclusive | inconclusive | hypermetropic astigmatism |
| 11 | intact | intact | normal | normal | cataracts corneal ulceration |
| 12 | intact | wax | mild | mild | blind L eye |
| 13 | wax | wax | mild | mild | cataracts, corneal opacity |
| 14 | opaque | wax | mild | mild | very poor vision |
| 15 | wax | wax | profound | profound | optic atrophy |
| 16 | wax | wax | profound | profound | glaucoma optic atrophy |
| 17 | intact | wax | mild | normal | hypermetropia |
| 18 | perforation | perforation | mild | mild | amblyopia |
| 19 | wax | wax | no cooperation | no cooperation | bilateral cataracts |
| 20 | no cooperation | no cooperation | ? mild | ? mild | strabismus |
| 21 | wax | wax | normal | normal | glaucoma |
| 22 | intact | wax | no cooperation | no cooperation | dense bilat cataracts |
| 23 | intact | wax | no cooperation | no cooperation | normal vision |
| 24 | intact | intact | profound | profound | primary optic atrophy |
| 25 | intact | intact | severe/profound | severe/profound | myopia |

Time is needed for familiarisation of the residents with the testing procedures, for repeat tests when co-operation has been problematic, for discussions with the key carets and for preparation of the plain English reports which require careful thought and effort from specialists who may be in the habit of communicating in writing only with others health disciplines.

It was agreed at the start of this project that implementation of advice would remain the responsibility of the primary consultants of the wards. Traditionally these have been consultant psychiatrists while the junior medical staff are registrars in psychiatry and clinical assistants. With the intention to transfer residents into the community, there have been major changes in medical staffing. The consultant psychiatrists have been transferred to clinics in the community and general practitioners from surrounding practices have been appointed to supplement the reduced clinical assistant cover. Most general practitioners therefore spend little time in the hospital and do not carry overall responsibility for medical care. It remains to be seen whether continuity of primary medical care can be achieved and whether this will lead to improved primary health care and appropriate specialist referrals.

The liaison speech and language therapist with one half day weekly, has found it necessary to restrict her efforts to just a few of the twenty-three wards. She has been concerned at delays in making referrals and offering of hospital ENT (otolaryngology) appointments. It has been difficult to ensure that key workers accompany residents and bring the appropriate information to consultations. The ENT consultant has suggested that the Project audiologists should be invited to supply and support the introduction of aids and this seems likely to prove acceptable to the NHS Trust. The Project optometrist already supplies and provides advice on spectacles, recommending referral to the opthalmologist for more complex disorders and for surgery.

When aids have been supplied, poor understanding of their use by the resident and lack of supervision by the key carer has led to their loss or damage in several cases. Active encouragement has been necessary to ensure that even the simplest measures are carried through. Perhaps the most important factor in the success or failure of the project with regard to each individual has been the interest, insight and permanence of the key carer and the relationship which develops between the resident and the key carer. We have been dismayed to find how frequently this relationship is broken by organisational changes. It is clear that a person who cannot understand his past and present health problems or recount these in speech is highly vulnerable to a change of carer. Arriving at a hospital clinic without someone who is able to provide a clear account of their past history and present problems, residents are unlikely to receive the help they need. The hospital administration is now responding by increasing therapy and training time for ward staff and residents.

Entering the health information from these 600 people into a relational database and learning how to present and analyse the data is a challenge for which our computer skills are developing gradually. Regular advice from an administrative assistant with wide experienced of databases would be of value. Because of the interest of caring staff and departments in the hospital and the community, we deal with ever-increasing requests for information which might be answered by a telephone 'health help-line' which could become part of the monitoring role. The database itself is the potential core of a permanent regional health register.

## *Comments and Recommendations*

Delivery of quality health care to multiply disabled people may be obstructed by certain attitudes which are common at the present time. These include:

1. ignorance of the brain disorders which lead to disability;
2. failure to understand that these may be prevented and treated effectively;
3. scepticism that this knowledge may benefit the individual and society;
4. fear of the responsibility of knowing, since knowledge dictates action.;
5. fear of the cost of heath care.

When these attitudes are allowed to dictate policy, the result is a system of containment in which it is tacitly agreed that while obvious health crises will receive treatment, underlying medical conditions will not be acknowledged.

In choosing to assess vision and hearing we selected the most obvious argument to demolish this illogical and unethical stance. Poor vision and hearing may be corrected in many disabled people and can be satisfactorily accommodated in others provided that it has been truly understood. The cost of such care is not great.

On the other hand, the cost of neglecting the vision and hearing of disabled people is very great. Failing eyesight and hearing lead to increasing dependence, distressed, 'challenging' and 'self-injurious' behaviours', unnecessary medications, iatrogenic illnesses, low morale and a high sickness rates among carers with inevitably escalating expense.

It is not only neglect of visual and hearing loss which carries these consequences. Failure to diagnose and understand underlying neurological and genetic conditions is also disastrous since each specific diagnosis carries possibilities for treatment and each has its own characteristic profile of impairments and skills within which therapists and carers must learn to work. Each disorder is associated with specific risks to be avoided or planned for.

By recording previous diagnoses and assessments in key areas of health, we have drawn attention to existing deficits in the programme of regular medical assessments for adults with learning disabilities and indicated the multiplicity of complex health problems which may coexist in one individual. The box summarises the anticipated outcomes of our project.

It is clear that people with learning disability are likely to require advice from a range of senior medical specialists in neurology, opthalmology, audiology, genetics, psychiatry, psychology, orthopaedics, paediatrics, nutrition and general medicine. Many medical specialities must therefore co-operate to provide the advice required by this multi-disabled population.

---

### Anticipated Outcomes Of Vision & Hearing Project

- Vision & hearing assessments achieved for all residents
- 'Plain English' reports provided to explain needs to carers
- Increased awareness of the value of accurate health advice
- Increased carer insight into how to look after health
- Establishment of a regional health needs database
- Development of realistic concepts supporting access to health care

---

The primary physician or general practitioner is competent to detect and treat a range of medical disorders, the strength of his position lying in the fact that he knows the whole family and its environment and can manage episodes of illness within this context. Routine annual medical examination by the general practitioner should detect such disorders as diabetes and hypertension. When complex neurological, genetic, psychiatric, nutritional or surgical problems are present which are beyond his or her competence, the general practitioner's role becomes that of gateway to specialist services (Kerr, Dunstan and Thapar, 1996).

Since learning disabled people suffer a high incidence of complex and multiple impairments which are easily overlooked on routine examination and because they cannot independently gain access to the appropriate assistance, it is clear that the provider must offer periodic specialist assessments in those areas of outstanding medical importance. In our view a record of health needs, of which such specialist assessments will be part, should be made for each person and reviewed at intervals of no less than five years.

There are several ways in which such a quality service can be achieved and providers of health care should be responsible for consulting with the full range of senior clinicians in order to decide how best the service can be integrated and monitored (see box) .

---

### Essentials for a Community Health Care Service

- Continuing instruction on health issues for carers, therapists & physicians.
- Habitual health surveillance by carats and professionals.
- Annual review and medical examination by the general practitioner.
- Community liaison nurses attached to specialist clinics.
- Routine provision by all specialists of plain English reports for carers.
- Automatic five-year specialist health assessments of mobility, nutrition, vision, hearing, communication, seizure, neurological and psychiatric state.
- Regional Health database linked to paediatric care.

---

However for this to be achieved, it will necessarily include several 'first-line' service elements:

1. a general surveillance system which registers all multiply disabled people, whether or not they have approached the health services. This system should be linked to the regional paediatric register.
2. primary medical care ( through general practitioner services)
3. a local disability services (with community nurses and therapists)

Any of these systems may accept the responsibility for co-ordinating the periodic specialist medical assessments. The family and the chief carer should be welcomed during the recording of needs and the specialist assessments, and invited to participate in decisions which follow. The general practitioner, the family and chief carer should receive a full copy of the completed assessment.

The hospital-based, specialist medical services which are most often consulted to advise intellectually disabled people will find it necessary to set aside extra time at clinics, provide additional staff and develop facilities to provide an effective specialist service. Special expertise may be most readily developed and most effectively used when it is concentrated in special units for advice on complex disabilities as has been done successfully by paediatric assessment units and a growing number of

'University Affiliated Programmes' (Welsh Health Planning Forum 1992). This is particularly helpful for people who require specialist advice from many departments since a single day in the unit can include several appointments with the same specialists as for the able population but with additional support.

Assessment of severe and complex epilepsies may require short periods of residential assessment for which a specialist unit has great advantages. Expensive equipment which must serve an entire region may be justified only if it is in frequent use in experienced hands.

Delivery of health care to the general public depends upon the affected person actively seeking help and explaining the present symptoms and how they have arisen. Adults with severe intellectual impairments cannot do this and as they grows older they are increasingly unlikely to have a life-long advocate who has known them sufficiently long or well to act as a substitute. Long term relationships, whether with family, friends or carers should be highly valued and protected. When a health specialist provides advice, a copy of this should be routinely provided for the chief carer - explained when necessary - as well as for the general practitioner.

This project has shown a need for continuous in-service health education for a growing number of carers from many professions including the families of multiply disabled people and the disabled themselves. In order to be effective in health surveillance and implementation of health advice, carers need to be well informed on a wide range of health issues There will be a growing need for a truly informative medical literature which can serve these groups of people and there will be an important role for a regional centre which can combine first-hand knowledge of the multiply disabled people in the area and their health needs with a service capable of teaching, advising on the development of services and providing library facilities and other resources.

## References

Kerr, A.M. (1994). Medical Concerns in people with severe learning difficulties: report on a vision week and symposium at the Royal College of Physicians and Surgeons of Glasgow, Scotland, 8-12 March 1993. *Journal of Intellectual Disability Research*, 38, 85-95.

Welsh Health Planning Forum (1992). *Mental Handicap (Learning Disabilities) Protocol for Investment in Health Gain*, Welsh Office. NHS Directorate, Cardiff.

Kerr, M., Dunstan, F. & Thapar, A. (1996). Attitudes of general practitioners to caring for people with learning disability. *British Journal of General Practice,* 46, 92-94.

McCulloch, D., Sludden, P., McKeown, K. & Kerr, A. (1996). Vision Care Requirements among intellectually disabled adults: a residence based pilot study, *Journal of Intellectual Disability Research,* 40, 140-150.

**Acknowledgements**
The author gratefully acknowledges the commitment and skill of colleagues in the project team: Tom Law and Aileen Campbell, Dr Daphne McCulloch and colleagues from the Caledonian University vision science department (optometrists), Barbara McLean and Elizabeth Coleman (audiologists), Elaine Newell (secretary), Susan Wallace (speech and language therapist) and Ian Crawford (finance). Ward staff have been helpful and interested throughout the project. Although therapy departments and the social work teams were unable to become directly involved, they have shown interest in the project and appreciation of the reports. Staff in the records department have been unfailingly supportive. Dr Bill Short and Clinical assistants, especially Dr Gavin Laird and Dr Nitze Pauleau have given all the support time allowed. The administration has provided a room and equipment for the project. Funding of the main project is provided by the Greater Glasgow Health Board and the Community Mental Health Trust and of the Health Watch pilot project by the Glaxo-Wellcome Medical Fellowship. The Medical Illustration Department of the Royal Hospital for Sick Children has prepared the illustrations for publication. The work was carried out at Lennox Castle Hospital.

**Alison Kerr** is Senior Lecturer in paediatrics of chronic neurological disability, University of Glasgow; honorary consultant in Community Child Health, Royal Hospital for Sick Children, Glasgow and in Learning Disability at Lennox Castle Hospital, Glasgow. Dr Kerr conducts the British Isles Rett Syndrome survey based in the Academic Centre, Gartnavel Royal Hospital.

**Contact Address**
Monitoring Unit, Academic Centre
Glasgow University Department of Psychological Medicine,
Gartnavel Royal Hospital,
1055, Great Western Road,
Glasgow G12 0XH
Scotland

# 5

## Meeting The Mental Health Needs
## Of The Elderly Person
## With Intellectual Disabilities

### Sally-Ann Cooper

The latter half of the 20th century has seen many changes for people with intellectual disabilities. Lifestyles have improved through the advent of care in the community, and access to medical treatments that used to be denied, for example the use of antibiotics to treat chest infections and surgery to correct congenital heart defects. This has resulted in considerable increases in the life span of people with intellectual disabilities. In the past, people with intellectual disabilities did not usually live into middle or old age, but now many can expect to achieve this. Life expectancy is greatest for those with less severe intellectual disabilities, who are mobile, female and do not have Down's syndrome (Jacobson, Sutton and Janicki, 1985).

With the closure of the institutions, and the move towards care in the community, elderly people with intellectual disabilities in the UK now live in a range of different types of residential settings.

- A few live alone in their own homes supported by care at home packages delivered by Social Services/care management, private or charitable organisations.
- Many live in residential care: these may be homes established to care for people with learning disabilities, such as Social Services hostels, private care homes, Mencap Homes Foundation homes, or homes established to care for elderly people, that is Social Services Part III homes, nursing homes and private residential homes for the elderly.
- A small number of people will live in re-provided community National Health Service homes for people with learning disabilities.

In any of these settings, elderly people with intellectual disabilities are likely to be in a minority. This presents a particular challenge to carers in identifying health needs when they occur. Carers working in services for elderly people are likely to be inexperienced in recognising and understanding the health needs of people with intellectual disabilities. Conversely, carers working in services for people with intellectual disabilities are unlikely to be experienced in recognising and understanding the health needs associated with old age because such services have traditionally been focused on younger people, with emphasis on development and skill acquisition.

The worst outcome of this might be that the health needs of someone living in a service for elderly people are ascribed to "it's just because she/he has intellectual disabilities", and therefore outside help is not sought for the person. Similarly, the health needs of a person living in a learning disabilities setting are ascribed to "its because she/he is elderly" and therefore again not addressed. It is important that the health services work together with social care providers in order to meet this challenge, through an educational process.

## When Is A Person Elderly?

The term *elderly* is one with which we are all familiar, but it does not have a precise definition in terms of population characteristics. The term conveys an impression of someone being a senior citizen, experienced and long-lived. Where services have been developed for elderly people, many have used an age cut-off to define elderly; this is often 65 years of age or older. Although such a definition is purely arbitrary, it does have the advantage of being precise and without ambiguity. However, in terms of a person's needs, some people who are younger than 65 years may have needs which are similar to the elderly group, whereas some people aged over 65 years can be more similar to younger people. This is just as true for the whole population as it is for people with intellectual disabilities.

As people with intellectual disabilities age, they develop needs which are age-related. In some special groups, these age-related needs occur at an earlier age than they do in the general population. An example of this is people with Down's syndrome, in whom it is well recognised that dementia is part of the behaviour phenotype (Oliver and Holland, 1986; Holland and Oliver, 1995). Some hold the view that most people with intellectual disabilities develop age-related needs more prematurely than other people in the general population.

The practical importance of these considerations is that the help offered to an individual has to be based on her/his needs, by whichever service can best meet those needs, rather than being "prescribed" on the basis of age. This will often require different parts of the health service to work together collaboratively, and will usually require people within different agencies (e.g. health and Social Services) to work together, along with any family members who are still involved, to the benefit of the individual.

A different approach is required when planning services. Effective planning requires these to be based on the level of need within the whole local population. In this way, services may well be planned for, e.g. people in particular age categories. However, operational policies must recognise the need for flexibility, when addressing the needs of an individual person.

## *Mental Health Needs Of Elderly People With Intellectual Disabilities*

### The Causes of Mental Health Needs

Many factors interrelate to cause mental health needs. Mental health needs are greater for elderly people with intellectual disabilities than they are for elderly people of average abilities (the general elderly population) or younger adults with intellectual disabilities. This is because they are vulnerable to all the risk factors for mental health problems that the general population are vulnerable to, the risk factors for mental health needs that are associated with old age, and additionally the risk factors that are associated with intellectual disabilities. Consequently, the mental health needs of this group are high. Some of these risk factors are listed in the box overleaf.

### Types of Mental Health Needs

Elderly people with intellectual disabilities have the same basic psychological needs as the rest of the population. These include being respected by others; a stable and caring environment to live in with companionship; opportunities for occupation and recreation; comfortable surroundings providing shelter, warmth, and food; having access to health and social care; and acknowledgement of, and attention to, individual cultural and religious backgrounds.

Additionally, they have needs due to their much higher rate of mental health difficulties, compared to the rest of the population. Researchers have examined the prevalence of mental health difficulties with three sub-populations. First, in people with intellectual disabilities aged 60 years and over, and living in institutions (Sansom, Singh, Jawed and Mukherjee, 1994). Secondly, in a population of people with intellectual disabilities aged 50 years and over (Patel, Goldberg and Moss, 1993). Thirdly in a population of people with intellectual disabilities aged 65 years and over, compared to younger adults with intellectual disabilities (Cooper, 1997a).

## The Causes of Mental Health Needs

**Risk factors affecting the general population**

- Physical causes e.g. family predisposition to mental health problem (genetic cause), carcinomas (such as breast), head injury, infections (such as hepatitis, glandular fever, encephalitis), progressive degenerative neurological disorders (e.g. multiple sclerosis).
- Psychological causes e.g. adverse circumstances during childhood, such as physical or sexual exploitation or abuse, neglect, lack of consistent parental figures or stable family background.
- Social causes e.g. life events, financial and housing problems, relationship problems, limited social network, lack of a confiding relationship.

**Additional risk factors affecting elderly people**

- Physical changes associated with age, e.g. onset of physical frailty, structural and functional brain changes, hearing impairment, visual impairment, medical illness and pain.
- Psychological factors associated with age e.g. loss of role upon retirement.
- Social factors associated with age e.g. bereavements and loss, reduced social networks, loneliness, reduced income.

**Additional risk factors affecting adults with intellectual disabilities**

- Physical causes e.g. behaviour phenotypes, epilepsy, hearing impairment, visual impairment, structural and functional brain abnormalities associated with some underlying causes of intellectual disabilities (such as brain biochemistry and Down's syndrome).
- Psychological causes e.g. disadvantages in early life that effect personality development (such as rejection, overprotection, repeated neglect, exploitation and abuse, being shunted around between different "care" providers).
- Social causes e.g. restricted income, carer stress, restricted social networks, lack of opportunities, lack of a close, confiding relationship, stigmatised by society.
- Developmental causes, e.g. becoming stuck in a developmental phase (such as head banging or establishing one's autonomy).

These studies show that depression and anxiety disorders occur in many people, and that dementia is particularly common. Pervasive developmental disorders (autism) are just as common in elderly as in younger adults with intellectual disabilities, as is schizophrenia/delusional disorders, and challenging behaviour. Sometimes challenging behaviour seems to start in old age. However, when this is the case, it is due to some other health need, e.g. the onset of dementia. Other mental health difficulties can also occur in elderly people with intellectual disabilities, although they are not common, such as mania and obsessive compulsive disorders.

Dementia occurs at a particularly high rate in people with intellectual disabilities. Amongst middle-aged people, much of this is accounted for by the high prevalence of dementia amongst people with Down's syndrome (Holland and Oliver, 1995). People with Down's syndrome may account for between a fifth to a quarter of the population in this age group. However, in old age, people with Down's syndrome form a very small part of the population, as most people with Down's syndrome do not yet usually live this long. Consequently, amongst elderly people with intellectual disabilities, dementia affects people whose intellectual disabilities are due to causes other than Down's syndrome. Indeed dementia occurs at a four times higher rate in elderly people with intellectual disabilities than in the age matched general population. This finding has been demonstrated in several research studies, but has received little attention (Cooper, 1997b).

## Presentation of Mental Health Needs

A key sign when someone develops mental health needs is that they change in some way. This may include them developing new behaviours which they did not used to have, or an exacerbation of their pre-existing maladaptive behaviours. Alternatively, previous behaviours cease which were part of their normal self. Other changes that may occur include the person developing new distressing symptoms or losing skills. If any of these changes occur in a person with intellectual disabilities, it is essential that they are referred for a health assessment.

Mental health needs present in different ways.

**Depression** If a person becomes depressed, for example, she/he may become more withdrawn than is usual, lose interest in the things that she/he used to enjoy, become irritable (less able to cope with little things that did not used to bother her/him; more likely to lose her/his temper), develop a labile mood, have less energy than usual, and appear to lose self care skills (probably as a result of losing interest and no longer being bothered about self care). The person may also experience a change in their sleep pattern (e.g. waking earlier than usual), a change in their appetite, may become more aggressive than usual and more anxious/frightened than usual. They may stop talking as much as previously, have episodes of tearfulness and seek more reassurance from their carers.

However, not all of these symptoms will occur in everyone who becomes depressed: some people will only change, for example in four of the above ways. Additionally, there are many other less common symptoms that can occur in a person if they are depressed. One person who develops depression may appear, at first sight, to be very different from another person who develops depression.

**Anxiety Disorders** A person who develops an anxiety disorder will experience episodes of feeling frightened and scared. This anxiety may occur out of the blue with no identifiable antecedent, or may occur as a result of something else (e.g. a knock on the door, having to go outside). Episodes of anxiety may be short (a few minutes) or prolonged (lasting hours) and may occur several times a day or less often.

Anxiety is often associated with symptoms that are due to overactivity of the autonomic nervous system, or changes in blood carbon dioxide levels secondary to a change in breathing pattern (hyperventilation). These symptoms including a pounding or racing heartbeat, chest pain, dry mouth (repeatedly wanting drinks), a lump in the throat (repeatedly swallowing), tremor, unsteadiness in walking, butterflies in the tummy or vomiting, sweating, flushing, incontinence and dizziness, amongst others.

If the anxiety symptoms occur as a result of something in particular (e.g. having to go outside), the person will usually try to avoid these situations, will try to escape from them when in the situation (e.g. by running away) and is likely to become very anxious in anticipation of such situations: this is often associated with aggression. When an elderly person with intellectual disabilities has an anxiety disorder, she/he will have some, but not necessarily all, of the above symptoms. Symptoms of anxiety may also occur as part of other mental health difficulties, such as depression and dementia.

**Dementia** This may also present in different ways with different people. The first indication that a person is developing dementia may include a loss of their adaptive skills, deterioration in their short-term memory, loss of other cognitive skills or a change in their behaviour. Examples might include losing the ability to dress themselves, or requiring more verbal prompts to complete this task, maybe putting clothes on back to front or trying to put both legs through the same hole.

Tasks that could previously be performed by the person might started to become only partially completed. The person might lose the ability to handle money as well as they previously did, or lose their skills in reading and writing. When put under pressure to complete these tasks, the person may become distressed and aggressive (a "catastrophic reaction").

Loss of memory may include not being able to recall the events of the day, whether things have or have not happened that day, and can result in the person asking repetitive questions, or repeatedly seeking reassurance on the same issue or failing to recognise people.

If the person becomes disorientated in time, they may get up in the middle of the night, insistent that it is time to go to the day centre. The person may also start to experience difficulties finding her/his way around. Someone who previously used to walk to the local shop alone, might get lost on the way, may forget the purpose of their trip out and so seemingly wander off. A person who used to find their way around at home, e.g. between the sitting room and bedroom, may lose the ability to do this. Being unable to find the way to the toilet may result in the person having episodes of incontinence.

Incontinence may also occur due to loss of skills (failure to recognise that the bladder is full or that voiding should take place in the toilet).

The person's ability to use judgement and make decisions may become impaired. They may develop dysphasia and dyspraxia. Concentration may become impaired. The person's sleep pattern often becomes reversed, i.e. awake at night and asleep during the day. The person with dementia often becomes apathetic and lacks motivation. Pre-existing personality traits may become more accentuated. Irritability can occur, as can anxiety, agitation and aggression.

Psychotic symptoms are also a common feature of dementia in people with intellectual disabilities, particularly the delusions that there are strangers in the house, that items are stolen from them, and visual hallucinations.

Physical changes also occur during dementia, including weight loss, the onset of seizures and regression in reflexes. The changes that occur during dementia are progressive, with the person becoming increasingly more dependent. During the final stages of dementia, a person will be unable to weight-bear, have incontinence of urine and their bowels, require feeding, be unable to talk, and unable to understand the events and speech around them.

**Psychoses**  An elderly person with intellectual disabilities may be psychotic due to long-standing schizophrenia/delusional disorder or due to the onset of a new problem.  Psychotic disorders are characterised by delusions (a false belief, which is held with conviction) and hallucinations (a perception which occurs without a stimuli).

Many types of delusions can occur, but often they are of a persecutory nature.  Many types of hallucinations can occur, but often they are auditory (hearing noises or voices when there is no-one there to account for them).  Other psychiatric symptoms occur together with the delusions and hallucinations: schizophrenia is associated with long-term progressive changes in personality and abilities, as well as acute episodes characterised by delusions and hallucinations.

## *Promoting Good Mental Health In Elderly People With Intellectual Disabilities*

The effective management of mental health needs amongst elderly people with intellectual disabilities requires collaboration between the agencies/ care providers, including carers (families, residential home carers), Social Services/care management and the health services.  Within the health service, community intellectual disabilities psychiatric services, mental health services for the elderly, and the primary health care team all have important roles to play.

### Education

A current obstacle to the provision of health care to elderly people with intellectual disabilities is lack of awareness of needs amongst carers (paid carers and families/friends).  Carers working in services designed for elderly people may, through inexperience, attribute health needs as being due to intellectual disabilities: carers working in services designed for people with intellectual disabilities may, through inexperience, attribute health needs as being due to old age.  In both cases, therefore, needs are accepted as chronic disabilities, rather than being a trigger for health referral for assessment and treatment.  This situation cannot be changed overnight but requires a programme of information and education to be made available to care providers.  Such a programme might be co-ordinated through, e.g. the specialist intellectual disabilities health service.  This might provide information both on the types of needs that elderly people with intellectual disabilities can acquire and how they can be met, and also the services that are available and how they can be accessed.

## Health Promotion

Health promotion can be addressed in an ad-hoc, opportunistic way. It may also be offered as part of a co-ordinated programme, targeting people within particular service provisions in a rolling programme, or identifying elderly people, e.g. through use of an intellectual disabilities register. Health promotion can include several components, including advice on a healthy lifestyle (e.g. diet, exercise, foot hygiene), optimising psychological well-being (e.g. advice and training in relaxation, recognising warning signs, and importance of relationships), advising on local screening provisions and facilitating the uptake of these. There is a particular role for community intellectual disabilities nurses in developing and implementing health promotion groups/ programmes.

## Health Screening

Health screening can be provided for both physical and psychological needs. The purpose of screening is to detect needs in the early stages, so that treatments can be offered before disorders become advanced or irreversible. General practitioners in the UK, through the primary health care team, offer annual screening to people registered with them who are over the age of 75 years. This includes people with intellectual disabilities.

However, general practitioners receive very little (if any) undergraduate, and no postgraduate training in intellectual disabilities. People with intellectual disabilities also form a very tiny part of their overall list size, and consequently it is difficult for the average general practitioner to gain experience in intellectual disabilities. For these reasons, it would be appropriate for the intellectual disabilities services to work together with general practitioners, to devise checklists/protocols that could be employed during these annual reviews. In view of the high prevalence of psychological and physical morbidity amongst elderly people with intellectual disabilities, the provision of annual health checks (as for the over 75's) would be likely to prove beneficial; as indeed may well be the case for younger adults with intellectual disabilities (see chapter by Hayward and Kerr in this volume). This is not an automatic provision in the general practitioner's contract in the UK, and so would require to be established as an additional service provided by the primary health care service, or the intellectual disabilities specialist health service.

People with intellectual disabilities should be encouraged additionally to make use of screening services that are provided for the general population, such as breast screening. However, because of the special needs of people with intellectual disabilities, they may require additional help to facilitate their use of existing screening services, e.g. a community intellectual disabilities nurse may prepare the person in advance with education about the need for the test and explanation about the procedure, and may help a person with limited verbal communication skills and limited understanding to actually cope with the test procedure itself (see Butler's chapter in this volume).

### Individual Care

An elderly person with mental health needs may require care from the intellectual disabilities psychiatric service or psychiatric services for the elderly. In part, this will depend upon the way that local services have been developed, and the expertise held within the different parts of the health service, which may vary from one part of the country to another. It will also depend upon the type of mental health needs of the individual.

Intellectual disabilities services have in the past focused on development and skills acquisition, whereas old age is a time of consolidation and coming to terms with loss. Elderly people form a very small proportion of all people with intellectual disabilities. Consequently, intellectual disabilities services still require further development before they can meet all the needs of this group. Psychiatric services for the elderly are experienced in meeting the needs of elderly people, but do not have experience in intellectual disabilities, pervasive developmental disorders, epilepsy management and how this interrelates with psychiatric disorders and behaviour phenotypes. Elderly people with intellectual disabilities form only a tiny proportion of the total elderly population. Consequently, the best care is likely to be achieved for a particular individual when the services work collaboratively, with the lead clinicians being identified on the basis of the individual's particular needs. This might mean, for example that care is provided by the intellectual disabilities service, with advice from the old age psychiatric service as required, or vice versa.

Some younger people with intellectual disabilities, who are under intellectual disabilities psychiatric care, might also benefit from advice from psychiatric services for the elderly, if they have age-related needs. As the number of people with intellectual disabilities who reach old age increases, it may become feasible for the larger centres to provide specialist services for elderly people with intellectual disabilities.

The health service can provide health assessments and devise treatment plans, but the majority of care plans will require multi-agency working.

Social factors interrelate aetiologically with mental health needs, and care plans may require manipulation of social factors.

Carers also need to be engaged in the process of devising care plans: they need to understand the reason for the plan and agree to it, as they are likely to play a vital role in its implementation, and hence in whether the care plan succeeds.

## Meeting Mental Health Needs

The management of a particular individual falls into two parts: assessment and treatment.

### Assessment

Comprehensive and detailed assessment is a mandatory precursor to treatment/care planning. If any elderly person is noticed to have changed in some way, or is thought to have mental health needs, this may require assessments to be undertaken by an intellectual disabilities psychiatrist, a psychiatrist specialising in the elderly, community intellectual disabilities nurse, community psychiatric nurse and/or therapists, e.g. clinical psychologist, occupational therapist.

The assessment will include undertaking detailed interviews with both the person with intellectual disabilities and their main carer. Information from these interviews will be collected on the change/needs that have been noticed, the severity and timescale of these. The presence or absence of a range of other psychiatric symptoms and maladaptive behaviours will be elicited. Any past mental health needs of the individual will be noted, together with the treatments which were and which were not effective. Drug histories should be collected, and also a record of past and present medical illnesses/ disabilities.

A record of the person's family health should be taken. A personal history is required, to ascertain the circumstances which have shaped the person's development, and particular difficulties to which they have been subjected, and in order to gain an understanding of the person's coping strategies. A social history should be taken, including details of recent life events, as well as social circumstances and relationships. Developmental history should include details of the underlying aetiology of the person's learning disabilities and their current developmental level/level of adaptive functioning, and past level of adaptive functioning, if higher.

A mental state examination and physical examination should be undertaken, together with special investigations. These are likely to include blood tests to check the person's full blood count, urea and electrolytes, liver function tests and thyroid function tests. Other investigations will be undertaken dependent upon the findings in the other parts of the assessment, e.g. other blood tests, urine tests, electrocardiogram, electroencephalogram, CT or MRI head scans (see chapter by Robertson and Murphy in this volume).

If the person has old medical case notes, it is important to check through these. In many cases, it is helpful to seek additional information from a carer from the past (this will depend upon the length of time that the person's current main carer has known her/him). In some cases, it is necessary for a longer period of assessment to be undertaken, e.g. to enable a functional analysis of behaviour. Occasionally, it may be necessary to undertake the assessment during a period of admission to an NHS unit. The information gathered in the assessments is integrated to formulate a description of the type of mental health problem that the person has, and a working hypothesis of the aetiological basis of this.

### Treatment and Care Planning

The treatment and care plan is dependent upon the formulation devised from the assessment. There are usually several components to the treatment/care plan, which broadly speaking, may be considered under the headings of physical, psychological, social and developmental interventions.

**Physical**    Physical interventions include general measures to optimise health by correcting any physical problems that have been detected in the assessment, e.g. treating thyroid disorders and anaemia, providing a hearing aid. Specific physical interventions may also be prescribed to correct psychiatric disorders, e.g. antipsychotic, antidepressant, mood stabilising and anxiolytic drugs, electroconvulsive therapy.

**Psychological**    Psychological therapies can be very simple, e.g. providing supportive psychotherapy through listening and explaining to the person with intellectual disabilities and their carers, or they may be highly complex.

Therapies may be aimed primarily at alleviating symptoms (behavioural psychotherapy) or at gaining insight into the origin of problems from which a person is enabled to change (psychodynamic psychotherapy). In elderly people with intellectual disabilities and mental health needs, psychodynamic psychotherapies are less often used.

Behavioural psychotherapies can be beneficial; these may include relaxation therapy and anxiety management although in people with severe intellectual disabilities, this will focus more on semi-hypnotic techniques, such as music, distraction, aromatherapy, massage, Snoezelen rooms, rather than progressive muscular relaxation and cognitive approaches.

Other treatment approaches include programmes of graded desensitisation for phobic anxiety, anger management, response prevention programmes and programmes to positively reinforce adaptive (as opposed to maladaptive) behaviours.

Approaches that may be beneficial when a person develops dementia include advising carers about the progressive nature of the disorder and hence to provide encouragement and prompts, but to accept new limitations and not to press the person to complete tasks she/he is no longer able to do, retaining skills through frequent use, applying routines and structure to the day to aid familiarity, reality orientation, e.g. using pictorial daily planners to guide and remind the person which part of the day it is and what happens when, putting pictures on doors to aid location of rooms and toilets, keeping a pictorial scrapbook of important people and events, using reminiscence groups as a means of recreation, socialisation and mental agility.

Listening to problems, talking these through and helping people to make sense of the events around them can be beneficial. Bereavement can be a bewildering as well as distressing experience for a person with intellectual disabilities, and is a common experience in old age. Consequently, bereavement counselling can often be of benefit. A person experiencing other life events and losses may also benefit from counselling.

**Social** Some needs can be met by social interventions. This may include programmes of occupation and recreation, environmental stability, providing a framework to recognise achievement, to respect an individual's culture and background, and to recognise the valuable contribution that each individual makes to society.

Encouraging the person's contribution to decision making, and helping them with self-direction and motivation can help.

Providing practical support to enable social networks to be developed and maintained can also be important measures to optimise mental health.

Many elderly people with intellectual disabilities have to share their main carer with several others, which limits the amount of individual attention that they receive. As people with intellectual disabilities do not usually marry or have children, their family networks are limited to siblings and nephews/nieces when their parents die. This also limits the amount of individual attention they receive and the likelihood of the person having a special relationship with someone. In times of greatest need, people may require considerable individual attention. Consequently, such an additional provision may be required when a person is depressed for example.

**Developmental**    Developmental approaches can be helpful in elderly people with mental health needs. Work on skill development can be used as a method of developing a relationship with a carer. This non-threatening situation may enable confiding to occur. Skill work can also help re-establish self-esteem and confidence following a depressive episode or anxiety disorder by building on a sense of achievement. It may also be used as a distraction technique.

The best clinical outcomes are usually achieved when treatments from the four categories listed above are used in combination rather than separately. The most appropriate treatments from the above list are determined from the assessment of need. The treatment list above is by no means exhaustive.

## Conclusions

People with intellectual disabilities are increasingly living longer. In the past, they did not usually live into old age but many can now expect to achieve middle or old age. However, special services have not been developed to meet the needs of this group. Those living in homes designed for elderly people may have mental health needs overlooked due to them incorrectly being ascribed to the intellectual disabilities while those living in homes for people with intellectual disabilities may have mental health needs overlooked due to them being considered to be a feature of old age.

Elderly people with intellectual disabilities have very high rates of mental health needs. This is because they are vulnerable to all the usual risk factors that affect everyone, but also have the additional risk factors that affect elderly people, and also the additional risk factors that affect people with intellectual disabilities. Anxiety disorders and depression are common, and dementia is particularly common. Challenging behaviour, schizophrenia/ delusional disorders and pervasive developmental disorders occur at a similar prevalence to that in younger adults with intellectual disabilities.

Meeting the challenge of providing mental health care for elderly people with intellectual disabilities requires education for carers, programmes of health promotion and screening, and individual treatment/care plans. These individual plans require an initial comprehensive assessment to formulate the type of mental health need, and its aetiological basis. Following this, the treatment/ care plans can be devised, and will usually require a combination of approaches; physical, psychological, social and developmental. Collaborative working between the different parts of the health service (intellectual disabilities service, psychiatric services for the elderly and primary health care), together with Social Services/care management, and families/care providers, is essential if effective outcomes are to be achieved.

## References

Cooper, S-A. (1997a). Epidemiology of psychiatric disorders in elderly compared with younger adults with learning disabilities. *British Journal of Psychiatry*, 170, 375-380.

Cooper, S-A. (1997b). High prevalence of dementia amongst people with learning disabilities not attributed to Down's syndrome. *Psychological Medicine*, 27, 609-616.

Holland, A.J. & Oliver, C. (1995). Down's syndrome and the links with Alzheimer's disease. *Journal of Neurology, Neurosurgery and Psychiatry*, 59, 111-114.

Jacobson, J.W., Sutton, M. S., & Janicki, M. P. (1985). Demography and characteristics of aging and aged mentally retarded persons. In: M.P. Janicki, & H.M. Wisniewski, (eds.), *Aging and Developmental Disabilities, Issues and Approaches*. Paul H. Brookes, Baltimore.

Oliver, C. & Holland, A.J. (1986). Down's syndrome and Alzheimer's disease: a review. *Psychological Medicine*, 16, 307-322.

Patel, P., Goldberg, D. & Moss, S. (1993). Psychiatric morbidity in older people with moderate and severe learning disabilities II: The prevalence study. *British Journal of Psychiatry*, 163, 481-491.

Sansom, D. T., Singh, I., Jawed, S. H. & Mukherjee, T. (1994). Elderly people with learning disabilities in hospital: a psychiatric study. *Journal of Intellectual Disability Research*, 38, 45-52.

**Sally-Ann Cooper** is Consultant in Learning Disabilities Psychiatry and
Clinical Director - Learning Disabilities at Rockingham Forest NHS
Trust. She is actively involved in research into psychiatric disorders in
adults with intellectual disabilities, especially elderly people and people
with Down Syndrome, and has published many research papers in these
areas.

**Contact Address**
Rockingham Forest NHS Trust
St Mary's Hospital
London Road
Kettering
Northants    NN15 7PW
England

# 6
# *Women's Health*

## Jenny Butler and Jane Tracy

During the second half of this century there has been an increasing awareness of the particular health issues faced by women. These issues are generally the same for women with intellectual disabilities as they are for the rest of the female population, however women with intellectual disabilities may have some specific areas of difficulty and concern.

In this chapter we will discuss a range of issues of particular importance for women with intellectual disabilities. They include:

- The development of social skills
- Issues relating to menstrual management
- Issues relating to fertility and sexuality
- Choices about contraception and pregnancy
- Symptoms of the menopause
- Preventative health strategies including routine medical review, cervical screening, breast checks, identification of cardiovascular risk factors and discussion of the effects of drug use including smoking and alcohol.

## *Basic Principles*

In looking at how we respond to women with intellectual disabilities and specific women's health problems it is important to remember the following guidelines:

- Women with intellectual disabilities have the same health needs as all other women and have the same rights as other women in the community to access relevant and appropriate information or treatment.

- Recommended treatment options should be the "least restrictive alternative", and always in the best interests of the individual. Whenever possible always include participation from the individual concerned in any decision making.

- Because of the very personal and sensitive nature of some women's health issues, respect and dignity for the individual should always be an important consideration. For example; whenever possible the woman should be able to choose to see a female doctor, have a female carer attend appointments with her, or to assist with her personal needs.

• Generally it is a good idea to work from the starting point of - "What if this was me/ or my daughter? What would happen and what would I like to see happen?"

• Carers and other professionals need to be mindful that their own personal and cultural values and beliefs do not infringe on their approaches to dealing effectively with women's health issues.

## Issues For Adolescents And Young Women

As a young woman approaches adolescence she will experience many physical and psychological changes.

Adolescence is a time of change and development for all young people. Young women, including those with intellectual disabilities, need to be well prepared to deal with the new challenges they will face in the transition to adulthood.

For young women with intellectual disabilities there may be particular difficulties that arise. They may not have the same opportunities in their daily life for the informal learning that occurs within peer groups of those without disabilities. Access to accurate and appropriate information may be limited, and for some, there will also be few opportunities for appropriate peer modelling. This may mean the young woman has restricted experiences to learn about the complex relationships and social behaviours of other adolescents. Therefore these young women may need formal and ongoing teaching about their bodies and appropriate social skills.

The following sections highlight particular issues and challenges that face young women at this time.

### Social Behaviours

During adolescence most young people move from relationships within same sex groups, to individual relationships with someone else. The interpersonal skills required are complex and young women with intellectual disabilities may feel confused, excluded and left behind.

As young women with intellectual disabilities grow up they need opportunities to learn and to practise appropriate social skills. Their cognitive difficulties may mean that they take longer to grasp these ideas than their non disabled peers. It is important to ensure that ample time is taken before adolescence begins to teach young women these skills.

Basic concepts important for the development of these skills include:

- **Private parts of their bodies**   Young women need a clear understanding of which body parts are considered to be private, and therefore only to be touched by the woman herself or by others with her express consent. In our society these private body parts include the breasts, genitals and buttocks.
- **Public and private behaviours**   Some behaviours are considered private and should only occur in private places. Behaviours such as undressing, toileting, the washing of private body parts, masturbation and sexual activity are included in this category.
- **Public and private places**   Someone's bedroom and the bathroom and toilet are considered to be private places. Private behaviours are acceptable in these places but not in others.
- **Protective behaviours** Young women need to acquire protective behaviours for their physical and sexual safety.  An understanding of the public and private body parts, places and behaviours, together with a clear sense of the woman's right to decide what she and others may or may not do with her body, are fundamentally important for her to develop appropriate protective behaviour skills. Many women with intellectual disabilities need some assistance learning about their rights and about specific strategies they are able to use when these rights are threatened.  Some women will remain vulnerable to abuse by others and will require support and care by those working with them to ensure that their rights are not violated.

Having a firm grasp of all these basic concepts will help women to develop and maintain relationships, and decrease their vulnerability to inappropriate approaches and behaviours of others.

### Risk Taking Behaviour

Many teenagers take risks for a wide variety of reasons. These include actions whereby:
- they tend to act spontaneously and impulsively,
- they have a belief that bad things won't happen to them,
- they wish to express their independence from their parents,
- they want to be like their friends and do the things their friends talk about and do,
- they want to impress their peers,

- they want to explore the world and their power to make their own decisions.

For adolescents with intellectual disabilities there may be additional problems in being able to plan ahead, foresee the consequences of their actions and think through the options available to them. They need specific and appropriate information about social situations and appropriate behaviours, for instance on how to handle peer pressure and about the effects of drugs on their bodies (including nicotine and alcohol). They need opportunities to express their independence and individuality in non harmful ways. They may need assistance in exploring different peer groups (through recreational clubs for example). They often benefit from opportunities to talk about their experiences and choices with someone whom they trust from outside the family.

## *Menstrual Management*

Most girls who have an intellectual disability begin menstruating at the usual time as their non disabled peers. It is very helpful to begin to prepare for menstruation in advance. How a young women feels about the onset of menstruation will be greatly influenced by the attitudes expressed by those around her. Understanding what will happen and how to manage her menstruation will avoid some of the difficulties that some young women and their carers face at this time.

The options available to young women with intellectual disabilities are the same as those available to all women. Most who are independent with toileting will have no difficulty when the correct use of pads is demonstrated and will be independent in menstrual management.

There is now a wealth of teaching material and information available to women, and those working with them, about the management of menstruation. The wide range of menstrual hygiene products available means women are usually able to choose one that suits their menstrual flow needs, and their ability to perform the manipulative hand movements needed to change pads.

Some women find the pads with large peel off paper strips revealing a sticky surface that can be applied to underpants is suitable for them. Others will find that continence pads, or pants that contain a pocket into which pads can be inserted, are easier to manage.

Specific instruction will usually be necessary and it is often helpful if this is accompanied by written material, drawings and videos that outline the steps needed to change and dispose of pads.

The success of any menstrual management program will, however, depend largely on adequate communication of the information and options available to a particular woman, and her level of interest, understanding and commitment. Ultimately it will be the enthusiasm and initiative of the women, staff and carers that will determine the level of any program's success.

Many women find it helpful to record the timing of their periods and any associated symptoms. This assists the woman in preparing for the onset of menstruation, and in understanding the changes in her body throughout her cycle. These records are also of value when medical advice is sought in relation to menstrual disturbances.

## Menstrual Disturbances

Like all women, women with an intellectual disability can have particular menstrual difficulties and the strategies to manage these are the same as those used for women without disabilities. If menstrual symptoms continue to cause problems after simple measures have been unsuccessfully tried, then medical consultation should be sought.

There are a number of medical conditions associated with particular causes of intellectual disability and these may, in turn, also cause menstrual disturbances; for example thyroid disease in people with Down Syndrome. There are also a number of medical conditions, including epilepsy and mood changes, that may be profoundly influenced by the hormonal changes of the menstrual cycle. These conditions require specific medical interventions and medical consultation is recommended if these are suspected.

## Heavy or Painful Periods (Menorrhagia)

There is great variation between women in the amount of blood lost in each cycle. Likewise the degree of discomfort experienced varies considerably. It is the effect of the period on an individual's quality of life that indicates whether or not intervention is required.

If a woman with heavy periods is experiencing difficulty with menstrual management she may:

- change her pads more frequently
- change the style of sanitary product used
- take period pain relief medications, many of which also decrease the amount of menstrual blood loss.

If a woman is experiencing pain on some days in her menstrual cycle she may find it helpful to:

- Be less physically active on those days

- Lie down and apply warmth to her lower abdomen when in pain
- Take period pain relief medications.

If symptoms continue to problematic medical advice should be sought.

## Pre-Menstrual Syndrome (PMS)

Pre-Menstrual Syndrome refers to the range of symptoms experienced by some women prior to the period. These symptoms relate to normal hormonal changes and may include mood swings, irritability, breast discomfort, bloating, food cravings, acne and fluid retention. For some women these symptoms are mild or are not noticed at all. For other women they can be extremely unpleasant.

The range of measures that may help correspond to the differing symptoms experienced by individual women. These include

* *Strategies to promote a feeling of general well being, particularly in the premenstrual period*

- A calm and supportive environment,
- A healthy high fibre and low fat diet,
- A regular daily pattern including exercise and good sleep patterns.

* *Specific strategies for premenstrual symptoms*

- Relaxation techniques,
- The keeping of a menstrual diary so the woman, and those working with her, can more easily understand and predict symptoms,
- Vitamin B6, B1, Evening Primrose Oil and other herbal preparations may be helpful for some,
- Medical consultation if symptoms continue to be problematic.

## Irregular Periods (Polymenorrhoea/Oligomenorrhoea).

A woman's periods are often irregular for the first few years after they begin in adolescence. If they remain irregular, or if they become so after a time of regular menstruation then a full medical assessment is required. This assessment may include the documentation of the cycle frequency and length, gynaecological examination and investigations.

For particular women;

- explanation of the irregularity may be all that is required
- hormonal medication to regulate cycles may be prescribed
- hormonal menstrual suppression may be considered

### No Period (Amenorrhoea)

A range of diseases and conditions, including pregnancy, may be associated with amenorrhoea. If a period is missed a medical consultation may be necessary in order to identify the cause.

### Menstrual Suppression

For most women menstruation is a normal and healthy part of their lives. For some, however, the suppression of the menstrual cycle will be an appropriate choice.

The circumstances in which this is may be considered are:

- Where the woman makes an informed decision to suppress her menstruation
- Gynaecological conditions e.g. endometriosis
- Medical conditions causing significant problems as a result of the menstrual cycle e.g.: certain types of epilepsy
- Where significant behavioural problems associated with the management of menstruation causes a serious negative effect on quality of life.

Menstrual suppression refers to the use of medications or surgery to temporarily or permanently stop menstruation. Hormonal contraceptive agents, both oral and injectable, can be used for temporary menstrual suppression. Endometrial ablation and hysterectomy are surgical methods used for permanent menstrual suppression.

In some cases menstrual suppression may result in lower circulating oestrogen levels. This in turn may lead to an increased long term risk of osteoporosis. Those using this form of menstrual management need to be aware of the potential risk and have it monitored appropriately by their doctor.

## *Sexuality*

Women with intellectual disability have the same range of sexual feelings and needs as women without a disability. Some will choose to be sexually active, others may not. Women need opportunities to discuss their feelings and the options available to them. It is important that women understand the rights and responsibilities involved in sexual activity and the consequences that may result from their decisions. Women also need appropriate information, education and skills in order to protect themselves from the unwanted consequences of sexual activity, and exploitation by others.

## Contraception

If a woman decides to become sexually active she will need to understand the contraceptive options available to her. Whatever choice she makes, it is important that she is aware of the need to protect herself against sexually transmitted diseases by practicing "safe sex" including sexual practices not involving penile penetration and the use of condoms.

Condoms may be used as the contraceptive method, but rely heavily on the knowledge and cooperation of the woman's male partner and this may be a disadvantage in some particular instances.

Spermicidal gels, creams and foams may be useful when used in conjunction with condoms but, when used alone, they have a high failure rate and are not recommended as a suitable contraceptive agent for most women.

The diaphragm is found by many women to be difficult to use and has a higher failure rate than most other methods. It's use also relies heavily on the woman planning ahead to ensure it's placement is absolutely correct every time she has intercourse. Many women, including those with intellectual disabilities, find it a difficult and unsatisfactory contraceptive method to use and it is therefore not generally recommended.

The combined oral contraceptive pill is used by many women. This method works best if the woman has a regular daily routine into which she can place her pill taking. This minimises the chances that pills will be forgotten. Short term side effects may include nausea, skin changes, headaches, mood swings and weight gain. For most women these are mild or non-existent and the pill is generally a satisfactory contraceptive method.

For some women the short term side effects of the pill are severe or unacceptable, for example the pill may cause a raised blood pressure, migraine or troublesome mood swings. Women may also be at a slightly increased risk of blood clots, heart attacks or strokes. The risk of serious side effects is small but all women should have a medical review before starting on the oral contraceptive pill. For women who smoke, particularly if they are over 35, another contraceptive method may be more appropriate.

The progestogen only pill is appropriate for some but requires very accurate pill taking and does not regulate the menstrual cycle in the same way as the combined pill. This pill has few side effects apart from irregular periods.

Some women choose the convenience of a three monthly injection of Depo Provera (an injectable form of progesterone). This method does not require remembering the daily pill and the woman can be assisted to have her injection regularly. Irregular periods, headaches and weight gain are the most common short term side effects of this method but for most these can be managed with simple measures such as analgesics and appropriate diet. After some months menstruation usually stops and this may be seen by some women as an additional bonus.

The Intrauterine Device (IUD) is an effective contraceptive agent, but has a number of significant disadvantages. The discomfort sometimes associated with it's insertion may be unacceptable to some women as may it's tendency to cause heavier more painful periods. There is also an increased risk of pelvic infection, with a subsequent risk of infertility. This method is not often felt by women with intellectual disabilities to be a suitable method for them.

### Permanent Methods of Contraception (Sterilisation)

Some women will wish to have a permanent form of contraception. In view of the lifelong consequences of this decision it is essential that *informed* consent is gained for any sterilisation procedure or that the decision for such a procedure be made through a formal guardianship application to the appropriate statutory body to ensure that the woman's best interests are paramount.

Regulations regarding consent and guardianship issues differ both between countries and within countries and the appropriate regulations must be followed.

There are three permanent procedures:

- **Tubal ligation**: This is a relatively minor surgical procedure to block the fallopian tubes. Failures rates from this procedure are very low but do occasionally occur. This procedure can be reversed, but the surgery required is long and complex and there is no guarantee of pregnancy. For these reasons this procedure should be regarded as a permanent form of contraception.

- **Endometrial ablation:** is the permanent removal of the lining of the uterus. There is no guarantee that menstruation will completely stop and this should not be relied on as a form of contraception.

- **Hysterectomy:** is the surgical removal of the uterus and/or ovaries. This is a major surgical procedure which results in permanent amenorrhoea and irreversible sterilisation.

The most common sterilisation procedure used is tubal ligation. For women with disabilities there has been a relatively higher rate of hysterectomy than in the population of women without disabilities as these procedures have been used for menstrual management as well as contraceptive reasons.

It is important to remember that women who have had sterilisation procedures will still need to learn about safe sex practices to protect themselves against sexually transmitted diseases.

## *Pregnancy*

Women with intellectual disabilities may want to become parents. They will need the opportunity to discuss the rights and responsibilities of parenthood and to explore relevant issues. For some women with intellectual disabilities and their partners genetic counseling will be an important part of this process.

Women with intellectual disabilities may become pregnant by choice or inadvertently. Women need to understand their menstrual cycles in order to know when pregnancy may have occurred.

Some women will wish to terminate the pregnancy for a variety of reasons. In this case she should be given opportunities to discuss her feelings, the options available to her. Termination of pregnancy is safest for the woman in the first trimester (up to 12 - 13 weeks) and so early identification of the pregnancy is important to allow adequate time for an informed decision to be made.

If a woman continues with her pregnancy she will need additional information, assistance and support throughout the pregnancy. Clear facts about the changes to her body and the ways she can care for herself and her baby through the pregnancy will be needed. Facts about the pregnancy and about children and parenting should be presented in an appropriate form and language. We develop our attitudes to parenting and to children through our personal experiences, likewise parenting knowledge and skills are acquired through observing the modelling of others and our own experience. Young women with intellectual disabilities may have had limited opportunities to directly watch family and friends in parenting roles. For example they may not have had the experience of baby-sitting younger children. Their cognitive difficulties and limited literacy skills may further limit their access to the knowledge and parenting experiences of others. Women choosing to continue with their pregnancy, and to therefore become mothers, will be likely to need considerable support in their ongoing role as parents.

## Menopause

Menopause , or the 'change of life', occurs at approximately the same age for women with disabilities as it does for the rest of the population, for most that means between forty-five and fifty-five years of age. It is a milestone on her path through life and most women will pass it without difficulty.

Women with disabilities need to be given appropriate information so they can understand the changes in their bodies, and carers should be alert to symptoms so they can arrange treatment for women who may not be able to seek it out for themselves.

The cessation of periods may occur quite suddenly, or after a time of menstrual irregularity. Most women have little or no discomfort associated with menopause, but for others may be other symptoms associated with the falling oestrogen levels at this time. These may include:

- vaginal dryness and painful intercourse
- hot flushes
- headaches
- extreme tiredness
- mood changes
- behavioural changes

In the long term, oestrogen deficiency has been associated with an increased risk of cardiovascular disease and osteoporosis.

Hormone replacement therapy (HRT) should be considered both to relieve the short term symptoms and the long term risks. For some women, with or without disabilities, the risks and adverse effects of HRT may outweigh the advantages and the balance needs to be evaluated for each woman individually.

### Osteoporosis

Osteoporosis (brittle bones) is related to the falling hormone (oestrogen) levels after menopause. When bones become brittle they are more likely to break, sometimes during only minor falls. Some women are at particular risk of osteoporosis and these include

- women with a family history of osteoporosis
- women who smoke
- women who are underweight
- women who have had low intake of calcium in their premenopausal years
- women who do not walk or do not take weight on their legs.

There are a range of things women can do to prevent osteoporosis. These include not smoking, eating a diet rich in calcium and in doing regular weight bearing exercise throughout life. Once osteoporosis has occurred there are various medications that can help. These include hormone replacement therapy and medications specifically targeted to the bones.

### Heart Disease

Women are more likely to have heart attacks after menopause and this relates both to the general changes of aging and to the falling oestrogen levels after menopause. Weight control, regular exercise and not smoking are the best ways to avoid heart attacks.

### Urinary Incontinence

Young women may experience some incontinence during pregnancy or after childbirth, but this problem becomes more common in the older age group. Women may be embarrassed, or may experience rejection relating to urine leakage and smell. There are a range of effective medical interventions available and a full medical evaluation is important.

### Life Events

There may be other significant life events occurring for particular women at this stage of their lives. For some, the death or illness of parents may lead to emotional distress, and perhaps to changes in accommodation. For others changes in daily routines associated with retirement or changes in day placement, may cause distress and confusion, and even social dislocation. These stresses may cause a range of somatic, behavioural and psychological symptoms. When symptoms arise in a particular woman these environmental factors must be identified and addressed in their own right, just as the hormonal changes must be evaluated.

## *Routine Medical Reviews*

Women with disabilities experience the same range of health problems as the rest of the population. Because some may have more difficulty describing particular sensations and symptoms regular health checks are particularly important.
Such checks may include:
- general health review and identification of health risk factors

- physical examination, including blood pressure monitoring and breast examinations ( and demonstrating the way a woman can examine her own breasts)
- cervical screening for those women who are or have previously been sexually active
- mammography for those over 50 years of age, or earlier if they are at an increased risk of breast cancer.

And discussion of

- Importance of regular exercise and healthy diet, with particular reference to iron and calcium intake.
- drug use, including smoking and alcohol
- health implications of unsafe sexual activity, and information about safe sex practices
- Importance of breast self examination.

**Psychiatric Illness**

Identification and discussion of the symptoms of psychiatric illness may also be difficult for someone with significant communication and learning difficulties. The same range of psychiatric problems seen in the general community are seen in people with intellectual disabilities but the ways these manifest may be somewhat different. Changes in behaviour noted by others, as well as symptoms reported by the woman herself, may be important indicators of psychiatric illness.

## *Conclusion*

Women with disabilities encounter the same wide range of issues throughout their life journey as do other women. The starting point in assisting them along the way is to see them first as women, and then to take their disabilities into account. For women with intellectual disabilities specific and appropriate strategies need to be creatively used to support them to acquire the necessary information and skills they need to make decisions about their lives and to take their place in the community.

## *Further Reading*

Consensus Statement. The prevention and management of osteoporosis. *Medical Journal of Australia*, 167, Supplement, July 1997.

Court, J. *You and Your Teenager*. Angus & Robertson. Sydney. 1995.

Curran, J. & Hollins, S. The Prevention Of Mental Illness in People With Learning Disability. In A. Kendrick, A. Tylee & P. Freeling (eds.) *The Prevention of Mental Illness In Primary Care.* Cambridge University Press. Cambridge. 1996.

Fegan, L., Rauch, A. & McCarthy, W. *Sexuality and People with Intellectual Disability.* 2nd Ed. MacLennan and Petty, Sydney. 1993.

Kaur, H., Butler, J. & Trumble, S. *Menstrual Management and Women with an Intellectual Disability: A Guide for GPs.* Monash University. 1996.

Kaur, H., Butler, J,. & Trumble, S. *Options for Menstrual Management: Resources and Information for Staff and Carers of Women with an Intellectual Disability.* Monash University. 1996.

Llewellyn-Jones, D. & Abraham, S. *Everygirl.* Oxford University Press. Melbourne. 1986.

Llewellyn-Jones, D. *Everywoman: A Gynaecological Guide for Life.* 4th Edition. Faber and Faber Ltd., London. 1986

McPherson, A. (ed.) *Women's Problems in General Practice.* 3rd edition. Oxford University Press. Oxford. 1993.

**Jenny Butler** is a teacher and educational counsellor who works in the Developmental Disability Unit at Monash University, Australia. She has extensive experience in service delivery and systems review. She now provides counselling and service consultancy on health, human relations and sexuality issues for people with intellectual disability.

**Jane Tracy** is a General Practitioner also working in the Developmental Disability Unit. She has previously worked in general practice and women's health, and now works exclusively in the disability area. She has a special interest in early intervention, inclusive education, medical education and in the barriers to health care encountered by people with disabilities.

**Contact Address**
Developmental Disability Unit
Monash University
Melbourne
Australia.

# 7

# Oral Health and Dental Care for People with Learning Disabilities

## Elizabeth Treasure, Barbara Chadwick and Richard Oliver

This chapter describes oral health and dentistry for people with learning difficulties. There are a very large number of topics that may be of interest to you. We have therefore described as many as possible but this inevitably means that there is not as much detail as you might like. The chapter falls into two main parts. The first section describes the common diseases of the mouth, and what broad treatment options are available. There are two major diseases, dental caries (decay) and periodontal (gum) disease. Both of these very common diseases are preventable. The second section describes the dental services available for people with learning disabilities.

## 1. COMMON DISEASES

### *Dental Caries*

Dental caries (decay) is an extremely common disease. At age five years 45% (O'Brien 1994) of children have at least one decayed, missing or filled tooth. By adulthood almost everyone has been affected (Todd and Lader 1991). People from more deprived backgrounds have considerably more decay as do people living in some parts of the U.K., notably in Scotland, Northern Ireland, the North West and Wales (Pitts and Palmer 1995).

#### Prevention of Dental Decay

*Frequency of sugar consumption* Dental caries is a disease where tooth substance is destroyed when bacteria in plaque produce acid from sugar in food and drinks. Sugar is present in many foods even baked beans and tomato ketchup so it is difficult to completely avoid it. Decay is largely preventable if food and drink containing sugars (e.g. biscuits, cakes, sweets) are only eaten at mealtimes. In between meals, fruit or bread and spread are a 'tooth safe' option. This reduces the frequency of sugar consumption and it is this reduction that prevents decay. Most people enjoy sweets but, it is a good idea to have a special time of the week for sweets;  for instance Saturday morning is sweet time and everyone can look forward to it!

Many people forget that drinks (e.g. pop and squash) can also contain sugar. Frequent drinks with sugar will also cause decay. Using feeding bottles as a comforter particularly at night may cause major problems with teeth. Ideally only milk or water should be placed in feeding bottles. Dummies should never be dipped in sweetened substances (e.g. jam or honey).

***Sugar-free medicines***   Many people with learning disabilities are on long-term medication. Where this is in liquid form it is important that this is a sugar-free variety if it is possible. It has been shown that prolonged use of sugary medicines will lead to more decayed teeth (Hobson 1985). Ask your doctor to prescribe sugar-free medicines and buy sugar-free varieties from the chemist.

***Fluoride***   One factor has been shown to prevent more dental decay than any other - fluoride. Where it is present at one part of fluoride per million of water, it leads to a reduction in dental decay of 50% (Murray 1996). However, in the United Kingdom there are a very few areas with enough fluoride in the water. The two main areas with enough fluoride are the West Midlands and Newcastle-upon-Tyne. If you are unsure whether your water supply is fluoridated your water company will be able to tell you.

Most toothpaste sold in the United Kingdom contains fluoride and this is a very important way of preventing decay. Tooth-brushing with a smear of toothpaste should start as soon as the teeth erupt. All children, until the age of 7 or 8, need to have their teeth brushed for them as they do not have the manual skills to clean their teeth efficiently. However, people with learning disabilities or anyone who is not able to hold a toothbrush may need help throughout life.

Fluoride drops and tablets can also be used. The latest recommendations from the British Dental Association are that they should be used when recommended by your dentist (see note). They are an effective way of preventing teeth decaying but it requires much effort to take them over many years.

### Prevention and Your Dentist

The most important part of preventing decay is through dietary control and use of fluoride as described above but your dentist can also help with extra preventive measures in the surgery. Your dentist will help by cleaning teeth and by teaching you how to care for them. The dentist may also apply fluoride using methods that are only allowed in the surgery.

***Fissure sealants*** The top of molar (biting) teeth are the parts of teeth most likely to decay because of the fissures. It is possible to fill these fissures with a plastic to stop decay starting in them. Each tooth takes about 5 minutes to treat but the tooth surface has to be kept very dry while it is being done. Sometimes it is difficult for people to co-operate sufficiently to enable an excellent sealant to be placed and it is better to have no sealant rather than a poor one which may leak and allow decay to start underneath it. They are only used for permanent molar teeth, i.e. second back teeth.

### Treatment of Dental Decay

The way in which dental decay is treated depends very much on the size of the cavity. In the early stages of decay, before a hole appears, it is possible to stop and even reverse the process, by applying fluoride. Regular check-ups allow your dentist to diagnose the decay early when it is easier to treat. Your dentist may ask you to apply fluoride by paying particular attention to a specific area as well as to attend for more frequent appointments. Often the speed at which a cavity is progressing is monitored by taking radiographs of the tooth.

Once a hole has developed the only way to treat the tooth is by filling it, as the hole will become larger. Eventually, the nerve of the tooth may be involved. At this stage the tooth either has to have the nerve removed or be extracted. If it is left an abscess may develop. Fillings do not last for ever and therefore prevention is preferable. Each time a filling is replaced it is bigger than the one before and the technique required to replace it becomes more complicated, e.g. it could be necessary to crown a tooth if much tooth tissue has been lost.

## *Periodontal Disease*

Periodontal or gum disease is a major cause of tooth loss in adults, but its prevention begins in childhood. About 8 % - 15% of the population are at risk of developing periodontal disease (Murray 1996) but unfortunately there are no tests available to identify who these people are. Therefore prevention is important in everyone. We do know that people with immunological deficiencies are more likely to be affected and therefore people with Down's Syndrome do experience more periodontal disease than other people.

Dental plaque, a white bacterial film on the tooth surface, can cause inflammation of the gums (gingivitis) if it is not regularly removed by tooth brushing. If a person has gingivitis their gums look red and swollen. Gingivitis is treated by improving oral hygiene practices.

If the gums start to bleed this may be a sign of early periodontal disease. If the disease is allowed to progress then the bone supporting the tooth is damaged and, over a period of many years, this may be to such an extent that the tooth can be lost.

### Prevention

Good oral hygiene practices are the best way of preventing gingivitis. Teeth and gums should be brushed thoroughly at least once a day (ideally morning and night) with a fluoride toothpaste. If you have to help someone brush their teeth it is easiest to stand behind them and support their head. Professional scaling and polishing from a dentist or dental hygienist is also useful. Smoking is likely to aggravate periodontal disease and hence should be avoided.

### Drug-related Gum Problems

Some drugs, e.g. epanutin (phenytoin), in combination with dental plaque, cause a hyperplastic change of the gums. The gums appear to grow and may even cover much of the tooth surface. If the drug is changed the problem usually resolves. Where this is not possible impeccable plaque control will minimise the swelling. In a few very severe cases surgical removal of the excess gum tissue is indicated.

## Trauma

Accidents to teeth are very common but can be troublesome to treat. Toddlers and young children are most likely to be affected but at least 16% by four years of age have damaged their front teeth (Hinds and Gregory, 1995). Two groups of children are more likely to break their front teeth; children with poor motor skills who are prone to falling and those whose front teeth stick out beyond their bottom lip.

Accidents occur on bicycles, in swimming pools, playing sports but also around school and in the home. In older people the cause of accidents changes with fights often involving alcohol use becoming much more common.

Children with non-accidental injuries (child abuse) often (approximately 50%) have facial injuries (Becker et al. 1978) and this possibility must always be considered when looking at a child with facial trauma.

*Self mutilation* Some people have conditions which lead them to damage themselves. This particularly distressing condition can be very hard to treat and is of particular relevance to dentists as often the person will bite or chew themselves. It is important to find someone who has experience of helping with this problem.

### Prevention

People who play contact sports should wear mouth-guards. The best mouth-guards are those which are made to fit your own mouth but your dentist will probably charge you to have these made. Children whose teeth really stick out should see an orthodontist to discuss the possibility of having the teeth moved using a brace.

### Treatment

Everyone who has damaged their teeth should see a dentist as soon as possible. For accidents which happened out-of-doors it is important that tetanus immunisations are up-to-date. All injuries need emergency treatment but also a prolonged period of follow-up because teeth can die after accidents and this may result in abscesses and pain if not treated promptly.

*First teeth* Treatment of injuries to first teeth will concentrate on making sure that the child is free from pain and that any damage to the second teeth is minimised.

*Second teeth* Second teeth which are knocked out of the mouth should be put back as quickly as possible. Anyone can do this. If the tooth is dirty wash it gently in water *but do not touch the root*. Make sure it is the right way round - match it to the tooth next door to check - and gently push it back into the root socket. Take the injured person to see a dentist who should fit a type of splint to hold the tooth in place. If you just can't manage to replace the tooth store it in milk and take the injured person and the tooth to a dentist as quickly as possible.

Teeth which are broken need to have the damaged surface covered as soon as possible to prevent further damage to the tooth's nerve.

The final type of damage is to the root and also to the ligament that holds the tooth in its socket. Often the tooth appears to be normal but a dentist should still be visited so that radiographs can be taken and assessment made.

## Malocclusion

The second teeth of many people grow crookedly into their mouths. Orthodontists are dentists who have specialised training in straightening teeth. They can be contacted most easily through your own dentist. Teeth can be straightened by using braces which may be either removable or fixed to the teeth. If someone wears a brace tooth cleaning becomes even more important and it is usually necessary to use a fluoride mouthwash to prevent the teeth decaying.

There is some evidence to suggest that children with cerebral palsy have a higher incidence of malocclusion, especially Class II Division 1 malocclusion where the upper front teeth project forwards. When this happens in conjunction with a habitual lips apart posture, the upper front teeth are in danger of damage if the child falls over or has an epileptic fit. Unfortunately correction of the position of the teeth using orthodontic appliances can only be achieved in co-operative individuals, and, if the lips apart habit remains, there must be some doubt that the corrected tooth positions will be maintained.

## Teeth And Teething

Babies are usually born with no teeth and the first teeth erupt into the mouth at around six months of age. These are usually the lower incisors. These are followed by the other incisors, then the first molars at around 12 months, the canine or eye teeth at 18 months and the second molars at 30 months.

The second teeth start to erupt at six years and are usually the first permanent molar that grows *behind* the last primary molar teeth. These teeth are often mistaken as 'baby' teeth yet they are very important teeth as they help guide the other teeth into position. First teeth start to be lost at seven years but the last baby tooth may not be lost until the child is 13 or 14 years old. These dates are guidelines only and there is much variation from these. Six months earlier or later is normal.

### Problems with Tooth Eruption and Teething

In most cases teeth erupt with no problems. However, occasionally they may cause local irritation which may keep children awake or cause dribbling. Usually gently cleaning the new teeth will help but occasionally sugar-free pain killers may be needed.

Two groups of people with learning difficulties may have specific problems with tooth eruption. People with Down's Syndrome may have missing teeth that never grow and their teeth may be slow to erupt. It is very probable that the dates described will not apply to these people. People with poor muscular control of their mouths e.g. some types of cerebral palsy may have teeth that erupt into unusual positions because the tongue and lips are unable to perform their usual function of 'fine tuning' the position of the teeth.

## *Pain*

### Signs of Pain

If a person has problems with communication it can be difficult for them to say that they are in pain. The following signs may sometimes indicate that pain is present: head rocking or even banging, hand sucking, moaning, dribbling, loss of sleep or appetite and avoidance of certain foods. The behaviour will disappear if the problem is sorted. Sometimes a behaviour improvement will be seen after dental treatment when it was not known that there was a problem with teeth.

What is often more difficult is in identifying where the pain is coming from as there are several areas around the mouth which can also hurt; these are ears, sinuses and tonsils. Pain from teething is unlikely before 6 months. Confusion is very likely between earache and toothache and it is always worth having a child's ears looked at if toothache is discounted. If a dental check-up can find no problems in the mouth it is often worthwhile visiting the doctor.

## *Dribbling*

Lack of control of saliva can be an embarrassment for the carer as well as the sufferer, especially the older and/or more cognisant individual. Research suggests that the cause is not an excess of saliva production, but a reduction in the number of swallows, and an inefficient swallowing mechanism.

In addition to the social effects, loss of saliva from the mouth can also lead to a need for more frequent change of clothes, increased risk of sore and chapped skin around the mouth, and, in extreme cases, dehydration.

Treatment for this condition may include alteration of posture (holding the sufferer's head up to prevent the saliva from running forwards out of the mouth), intensive speech therapy, prescription of certain drugs, surgery to the salivary glands and their ducts, or provision of a special orthodontic plate called a Palatal Training Appliance. None of these methods can guarantee 100% success, and sometimes will provide only temporary and partial relief of the problem. Some people may be unsuitable for medical or behavioural reasons for one or other of these approaches to treatment.

Most clinicians will not prescribe drugs, as, in addition to drying up the flow of saliva, they will also dry up other important secretions such as tears and the lubricating fluid in the lungs. There is also a greatly increased risk of developing decay in the teeth when the mouth is dry.

## 2. DENTAL SERVICES

There are several reasons why people with learning disabilities merit special concern for dental care. The oral health of some may be different to their normal peers, e.g. people with Downs Syndrome have an increased prevalence of gum disease. The prevention of dental disease may be more important for some groups, e.g. the effects of bacteria on some heart conditions are very serious. Finally, the treatment that can be carried out may need to be modified according to the capabilities, co-operation and wishes of the person, their family or carers.

## *Behaviour Management*

Most studies have shown that the majority of people with learning difficulties can be examined and treated in the dental surgery with the rest of the family in the usual way. Little special equipment is required, although good access and ramps for wheelchairs are important for some groups.

What all people with disabilities need is comprehensive preventive care as early as possible. Like all people they may fear the unknown and new situations are always challenging. Short regular visits to a friendly dentist for advice and preventive care can give confidence to the child, the carers and the dentist.

If fillings are needed the ability of an individual patient to cope depends on their understanding and age. For some groups of people with learning difficulties this means that techniques usually used for young children may still be useful into the teenage years and beyond. Many people do not know what dental treatment involves and this can make them anxious. **Tell-show-do** is one way to help.

The dentist **explains** what they are going to do in simple language, **demonstrates** the procedure e.g. polishing a finger with a slow moving drill, and then **carries out** the task. This process of getting used to the dental environment or **acclimatisation** may take a number of short visits. Many dentists find that having the parents or carers in the surgery can be helpful as well. Parents and carers can also be used as **models** to help explain treatment, e.g. the dentist may examine a parent while the child watches to demonstrate what is going to happen, or videos of other people being successfully treated can be used.

For many people with learning difficulties dental treatment can be carried out successfully with a little time and patience. However, for a few patients treatment can only be carried out asleep. In such cases specialist centres able to offer general anaesthetic facilities are required. It is of course important to ensure that regular reviews and visits for preventive advice such as tooth-brushing still take place.

## How to Find a Dentist

If you have problems finding a dentist phone your local health authority who have a list of all dentists in the area. They will also have details on location and facilities offered such as if the practice is located on the ground floor of a building and is accessible to people with wheelchairs. Personnel recommendation is often the best way of finding a dentist who has particular skills in working with people with learning disabilities. It is very likely that this dentist will work in the hospital or community dental service.

### Paying for Dental Care

Dentistry provided in hospitals or in the community dental service is free although a charge may be made for dentures. National health service dentistry provided in general dental practice is free for people on low incomes and children under the age of 19. Dentists in practice will charge for patients who they are seeing privately. Always ask whether you are being treated as a private patient or as a national health service patient.

### General Dental Practice

Most people are treated in general dental practice. Dentists who work here are paid on the amount of work they do and sometimes are unable to spend the necessary time to provide care for people whose treatment takes longer. Most dentists will treat some patients with learning disabilities and certainly people with mild problems should be able to be seen here.

### Community Dental Service

In the community dental service dentists are paid a salary and are not so restricted by time. Community dental services have as their prime function the role of providing dental care for people who have difficulty in receiving it from elsewhere. Community dental services will have links with special schools and also with Day Centres. They employ dentists and hygienists who want to work with people with learning disabilities and who have developed special skills in doing so. In many parts of the country they will have specialised facilities and access to general anaesthetic sessions. The community dental service usually works closely with the hospital service when planning the care of people with learning disabilities.

Ask at your local health centre if you have trouble contacting them or look in the phone book.

### Hospital Dental Services

Many hospitals have consultants in oral surgery and in orthodontics. Some also have consultants in restorative dentistry. There are also dental hospitals in the largest cities in the country albeit only 14 in all. These exist primarily to train dental students and auxiliary staff but also provide care to people. It is probable that there will be people there with particular skills and interests in this area. You need to be referred to a hospital by your own doctor or dentist.

## *References*

Becker, D. B., Needleman, H.L. & Kotelchuck. M. (1978). Child abuse and dentistry; orofacial trauma and its recognition by dentists. *Journal of the American Dental Association,* 97, 24 - 28.

Hinds, K. & Gregory, J.R. (1995). *National Diet and Nutrition Survey Volume 2: Report of the dental survey.* London: HMSO.

Hobson, P. (1985). Sugar-based medicines and dental disease. *Community Dental Health*, 2, 57 - 62.

Murray, J., (ed.) (1996). *The Prevention of Dental Disease.* Oxford: Oxford University Press.

O'Brien, M. (1994). *Child Dental Health in the UK, 1993.* London: HMSO.

Pitts, N. B. & Palmer, J.D. (1995). The dental caries experience of 5-year-old children in Great Britain. Surveys coordinated by the British Association for the Study of Community Dentistry in 1993/94. *Community Dental Health,* 12(1), 52-58.

Todd, J. E. & Lader, D. (1991). *Adult Dental Health 1988 United Kingdom.* London: HMSO.

**Note:**

Fluoride supplement doseage; a policy statement by BDA, BSPD and BASCD. *British Dental Journal* , 182, 6 - 7.

**Authors**

The authors of this chapter all work in the Division of Dental Health and Development at the Dental School of the University of Wales College of Medicine in Cardiff.

**Elizabeth Treasure**  is Senior Lecturer in Dental Public Health and Consultant with Cardiff Community Health Care NHS Trust. She has researched the dental health needs of people with learning difficulties, worked in the Community Dental Service providing care to people with learning difficulties.

**Barbara Chadwick** is Senior Lecturer in Paediatric Dentistry and Consultant with the University Dental Hospital NHS Trust. She provides care to many people with learning difficulties and has a particular interest in behaviour management techniques.

**Richard Oliver** is Senior Lecturer in Orthodontics and Consultant with the University Dental Hospital Trust. He has treated a large number of people with dribbling disorders. He is particularly interested in the management of facial deformity. He is responsible for running a service for babies with cleft lip and palates.

**Contact Address**
The Dental School
Heath Park
Cardiff CF4 4XY
Wales

# 8

# *Sleep Disturbance: A New Understanding*

## Colin A. Espie

The term "quality of life" is widely used in care planning for people with intellectual disabilities. Although it is a concept which is difficult to define precisely, it certainly has to do with the benefits associated with how people spend their time. Since most people spend around one third of their lives in bed, the importance of sleep as a contributory factor to "quality of life" should not be overlooked. Sleep is a highly valued state and there are important relationships between the night and the day. For example, people perform at their best and are in a better frame of mind after "a good night's sleep". There is no reason to believe that the needs of people with learning disabilities are any different. In fact it could be that sleep is particularly important for people who have fundamental difficulties with concentration, with learning, and sometimes with emotional and behavioural expression.

This chapter is divided into two sections. Firstly, normal sleep patterns will be described. Consideration will be given to the nature of sleep, its importance, the amount of sleep that people need and how sleep changes with age. Particular consideration will be given to sleep patterns of people with intellectual disabilities.

Secondly, disorders of sleep will be introduced. Classification systems used in sleep medicine will be explained and, problems which are common in people with intellectual disabilities will be discussed. Emphasis will be placed upon treatment strategies which are *non-pharmacological*. These will be discussed and illustrated.

An attempt has been made to keep the text as readable as possible. Those references which do appear are to important papers or books which will provide the reader with further information.

## *An Overview Of Sleep Patterns*

### Characteristics of Sleep in the General Population

What is sleep? It is tempting to think that sleep is just the absence of wakefulness. However as William Dement, the great sleep researcher has suggested, sleep is more like a stationary car with its engine running, than one which is garaged for the night. Sleep is a very important time when a great deal happens. Although we switch off our light at bedtime, we are not switching ourselves off. In fact throughout the night there are different types of sleep (known as stages). There are four stages of orthodox or normal sleep. Stages 1 and 2 are "lighter" sleep and stages 3 and 4 "deeper". Deep sleep is particularly concentrated during the first couple of hours of sleep and light sleep is more common during the second half of the night. The stage of sleep when dreams tend to occur is known as rapid eye movement (REM) sleep. Dreams are not usually a sign of emotional disturbance, although some may be disturbing. Sleep stages 1-4 and REM sleep occur in a cyclical pattern across the night.

### Why is Sleep Needed?

The body provides signals for when to sleep and how much to sleep. The natural state is for sleep to be regularly patterned night to night. The 'body clock' which controls sleep and wakefulness follows what is know as a circadian rhythm, also regulated by natural light. When everything is going well, there is an equilibrium or balance in circadian rhythms.

Sleep is necessary both for physical and mental development and recovery. Amino acids which form the basis of protein, and important hormones are produced during sleep to rebuild the body. The harder the body works, the more the need to sleep. The same is true for the mind. However, it is not just to do with giving the mind a rest. The brain continues to work hard since information and learning is processed and stored in memory during sleep. Research has shown that REM sleep is particularly important for information processing and that deep sleep facilitates physical restoration.

### How Much Sleep?

This is probably the most commonly asked question! Unfortunately, there is not just one answer because the amount of sleep a person needs varies depending on age and stage in life, and on what s/he is doing. Sleep also varies from person to person, just in the same way as people who are in other ways similar, may have quite different shoe sizes.

The average sleep for an adult is seven or eight hours but it is quite normal to have less or more than this.

Some people can manage on as little as four hours. Amount of sleep does change throughout the life cycle. Infants and young children sleep for very lengthy periods. Here, stage 3 and 4 (deep) sleep and REM sleep are particularly plentiful, associated with physical growth and the acceleration in learning in younger years. Adults have less deep sleep and older adults sleep much less than younger adults, have more broken sleep with micro-arousals and wakenings, and they have a greater proportion of light sleep, especially in the second half of the night.

Therefore, it is clear, that individual sleep requirements vary and also change across the life span. (See Horne (1990) for more information on the nature and functions of sleep).

## Characteristics of Sleep in People with Intellectual Disabilities

### Limited Information

The sleep patterns of people with intellectual disabilities have not been widely studied. However, there is research evidence to strongly suggest that their sleep is significantly different from that of the general population. Before going any further it is important to stress that the term "intellectual disabilities" describes a wide range of disorders and syndromes, and severities of mental disability. Clearly, there is a danger of generalisation. The importance of assessing the individual and considering his or her particular sleep pattern, at a particular point in time, cannot be stressed too highly.

### Sleep Stage Differences

There are a number of research findings which have consistent support. The first is that people with intellectual disabilities have significantly reduced REM sleep. In one recent study we found that only 12 out of 28 people studied had measurable REM sleep, using sleep EEG (the electroencephalogram measures electrical activity in the brain during sleep). Furthermore, the total amount of REM was diminished compared with the normal population, even when it did occur.

A second distinguishing feature is the high level of what we have called indiscriminate non-REM sleep. Their sleep typically lacks the defining characteristics which permit conventional staging (into stages 1, 2, 3 and 4). For example, there is a relative absence of K-complexes and sleep spindles, which are characteristic of normal stage 2 sleep. Such differences in the 'architecture of sleep' are more pronounced in people with more severe intellectual impairment, presumably due to greater brain damage.

A third important factor for many people is increased daytime sleep tendency. People with intellectual disabilities appear prone to daytime naps. There may be both biological and environmental reasons for this. Biological factors include a poorly organised circadian rhythm, damage to arousal centres in the brain, and sedating medications. Environmental factors include lack of stimulation and dull or monotonous routines. (See Espie et al; in press).

### Influence of Care Practices

There is also evidence that people with intellectual disabilities spend longer in bed than would people of similar age from the general population. We have found that carers significantly overestimate the amount of time which people with learning disabilities actually sleep. In a group of adults (average age of 31 years), carers estimated that clients had slept 505 minutes on the study night, compared with 444 minutes as recorded by sleep EEG. (Espie et al, in press). Such an over-estimation of sleep is interesting (as normally people underestimate) and it may also be reflected in an over-estimation of sleep requirement.

Perhaps carers misperceive their own sleep needs. It is understandable also that many carers require respite. Indeed respite care is an integral part of most services. Quiet wakefulness and sleep provide readily accessible forms of respite, particularly for more compliant, passive or multiply handicapped individuals. Perhaps carers use the bed as an informal respite environment. However, putting people to bed may cause either wakenings during the night, or excessive daytime sleepiness since oversleeping tends to lead to a break down in the circadian rhythm. This can foster a pattern of napping and waking across the 24 hours.

A further difficulty arises in group living environments where sleep and wake patterns may be set for administrative reasons. For example, it is common practice for staff working from early afternoon until mid/late evening to have responsibility for preparing people for bed. Typically, this involves having people in night clothes relatively early in the evening. We have found that adults with profound intellectual disability are put to bed on average at 9.20pm and spend on average 10 hours and 40 minutes in bed. Even in small group living, scant attention may be paid to individual variability in sleep requirements both at the onset and offset of sleep. In circumstances where a staffed house has only one or two people on duty in the early morning, it may be necessary to begin to get some people out of bed very early (and others late) in order to have everyone prepared for the day.

## Classification of Sleep Disorders

The International Classification of Sleep Disorders diagnostic and coding manual sub-divides sleep disorders into dyssomnias, parasomnias and medical/psychiatric sleep disorders (American Sleep Disorders Association, 1990).

The most common *dyssomnia* is insomnia, that is a difficulty initiating or maintaining sleep. This category also includes hypersomnia (over-sleeping), sleep apnoea (a sleep related respiratory disorder), and disorders of the circadian rhythm, (where sleep is out of phase with night-time).

The more common *parasomnias* are sleep walking, sleep talking and night terrors. These tend to be deep sleep phenomena which is why it is very difficult to rouse, for example, a child from a night terror compared to a nightmare, which occurs in REM sleep. Both medical and psychiatric disorders can be associated with sleep disorder and a variety of drugs affect sleep adversely. (See Shapiro (1993) for a helpful review).

## Sleep Disorders In People With Intellectual Disabilities

### Common Sleep Disorders

Although people with intellectual disabilities can experience the full range of sleep disorders, there are few systematic studies identifying exactly how common (prevalent) each disorder is. Prevalence studies will always be hampered by the fact that sleep disorder is usually self-reported in the general population. The *experience* of sleep and its daytime consequences are the primary features of complaint. Communication difficulties restrict such reporting by people with intellectual disabilities and carer concerns are inevitably indirect, reflecting "management" difficulties. The likelihood is that many sleep problems pass undetected and untreated, others present as emotional/behavioural problems, and most will be greatly affected by the carer's perspective.

In spite of these difficulties, sleep disturbances are major sources of concern in practice, both amongst children and adults. Night settling difficulties, problems establishing a stable sleep pattern, sleep walking and night terrors, nocturnal seizures, sleep apnoea and daytime sleepiness are all priorities for assessment and treatment.

### Assessing Sleep Disorders

Before considering how to manage sleep problems it is important to consider sleep assessment. The basis for any sound diagnosis and subsequent intervention has to be good quality information.

It is important, firstly, to obtain a good_*sleep history* i.e. to establish what type of sleep disorder is problematic, how sleep difficulties have developed over time, onset factors, periods of improved sleep, previous treatment strategies and their effectiveness, etc. There are questionnaires which can be helpful here (e.g. Simonds and Parraga, 1982).

The current *sleep pattern* must also be assessed. The most reliable method is the sleep EEG but this will seldom be available other than for diagnostic purposes (e.g. apnoea, narcolepsy).

Full polysomnography (PSG) involves measurement of other physiological functions including respiration, heart rate and muscle tone. PSG, however, is not suitable for reviewing sleep pattern on a night-to-night basis or for continuous monitoring across a treatment phase.

Wrist actigraphs are sensitive movement meters which can yield some objective information on sleep pattern without overnight admission to a sleep laboratory. They are minimally intrusive, and recent models are well tolerated.

Sleep Diaries comprise information on the main sleep parameters (bedtime, time to fall asleep, number and duration of wakenings, rising time, total time asleep). These can be completed in simplified form by more able clients, or, more usually, by carers. There are published examples of such sleep Diaries (e.g. Espie, 1991)

A final aspect of assessment concerns *daytime functioning.* The daytime impact of sleep impairment may be considerable, and it is important to establish specific associations where they exist. Daytime napping can be incorporated into the Sleep Diary, since daytime sleepiness may be important diagnostically. Of course, daytime may also influence night-time i.e. it is a two way process. Behavioural analysis provides a useful framework for addressing daytime difficulties.

## *Managing Sleep Disorders*

### Night Settling and Waking Difficulties

These are relatively common in childhood, not least in children with intellectual disabilities. The child experiences sleeplessness and distress at bedtime, or when awakening, and does not spontaneously settle. The presentation may reflect separation anxieties in the child and/or parent. This may be regarded as a developmentally normal phenomenon which has not been outgrown. Maintaining factors are varied and can include concern over the child's health, phobic anxiety (e.g. of the dark, isolation) and secondary gain (the behaviour is reinforcing for one or more of those involved). In most cases there is clear habit formation and a cyclical pattern of failed attempts to settle and rising from bed. These children often end up sleeping with a parent and this "arrangement" can extend into adulthood.

Lyn Quine has outlined an effective treatment programme for such problems. (Quine, 1993; 1997) which is described in the box below.

---

### *Overcoming Night Settling Problems*

1. Identifying the problem and its cause. (Getting a clear description, recognising factors which contribute).

2. Specification of appropriate bedtime by parents. (Having clear agreed goals).

3. Introduction of a bedtime routine. (Establishing consistency).

4. Avoiding over-stimulation before bedtime. (e.g. quiet, enjoyable routines).

5. Teaching the child to relax to a specific cue (e.g. music or a bedtime story).

6. Gradual distancing of parent from the child's room. (Reducing physical contact in stages).

7. Rewarding appropriate bedtime behaviour. (Celebrating success, rewards for settling).

8. Dealing with waking problems. (Repeating 5,6 and 7).

---

There is also considerable evidence that parents of children with severe sleep difficulties become significantly stressed. It is important, therefore, to provide support to them for their needs and also encouragement in persisting with the treatment programme for the sleep disorder.

## Poorly Established Sleep Patterns

It is an interesting fact that most people who sleep poorly also at times sleep well. That is, there is night to night variability in the pattern and quality of sleep. This is typical of insomnia and leads to considerable concern and frustration. Sometimes attempts are made to compensate for the previous poor sleep by trying to sleep for longer on subsequent nights. Unfortunately, this usually makes sleep worse!

The concept of sleep efficiency is particularly useful here. This is the ratio of time slept to time spent in bed, expressed as a percentage. Therefore, six hours sleep out of nine spent in bed equates to 67% sleep efficiency. This is a useful starting point for treatment since efficiency can be increased either by *increasing the numerator* or *decreasing the denominator* of the ratio. Clearly, the latter may be an option since, as previously mentioned, people with intellectual disabilities can spend excessive amounts of time in bed and sleep less than carers anticipate. We have devised a programme, "sleep scheduling treatment" for inefficient and highly variable sleep patterns which has ten elements (see box opposite).

Clinical psychologists can often help in planning interventions for night settling/insomnia problems.

## Parasomnia

These are slow wave (deep sleep) phenomena and have been described earlier. They commonly first present during childhood and there may be a family history of others experiencing similar difficulties. Parasomnias can be regular or recurring disorders and can re-emerge or get worse at times of life change or stress. In this sense they may be useful indicators of emotional and social functioning. Interventions aimed at dealing with *sources* of anxiety and concern can be very effective.

There is little advantage in attempting to waken a sleep-walker or someone in the midst of a night terror. Indeed, active intervention can make agitation and distress worse, not only for the client but also for the carer. Rather, a reassuring approach is recommended, whilst ensuring that any potentially dangerous activities (e.g. walking downstairs) are supervised or avoided. The majority of parasomniacs do not recall these episodes in the morning.

# Sleep Scheduling Treatment

1. Establish morning rising time as a set "anchor" time, convenient to day time activities. (7 days per week initially).

2. Calculate average night time sleep length over 10 nights (as indicative of sleep requirement).

3. Subtract average sleep length from morning rising time. (e.g. if the average sleep of an adult is 8 hours and rising time is 7.30 a.m. then 7.30 less 8 hours equals 11.30 p.m.)

4. Establish a "threshold time" for going to bed which is no more than 30-45 minutes prior to the calculated time. The aim is to achieve around 90% sleep efficiency. (In the above example this would mean the threshold time was around 10.45 to 11.00 p.m.)

5. Upon reaching the threshold time, monitor the client's "sleep readiness", (assisting him/her to bed when he/she seems "sleepy tired", but not before.)

6. Adjust the threshold time if 90% sleep efficiency is achieved regularly and if the client is commonly sleepy, prior to the threshold time. (Changes in threshold time can be made at the rate of 15 minutes per week but should not continue if the client does not sleep right through the night.)

7. Plans must be made to consider how best to manage the evening period, which may now be longer. (Carers still require "respite" and assistance in planning quiet activities).

8. Try to avoid the client napping during daytime or evening prior to the threshold time. (Clients will sleep better if occupied and stimulated during the day).

9. Avoid recovery sleep to compensate for previous "poor" nights. (Try to establish consistency).

10. Persist with this programme for several weeks since it will take time for a new sleep pattern to be firmly established. (Continue with encouragement and support).

Carers also often require education and reassurance since night terrors, in particular, can have an hallucinatory quality and be distressing to observe (See Shapiro; 1993).

## Nocturnal Seizures

These are mentioned briefly since they can be disruptive of sleep for the client, but also for carers. Some people also have seizures when they lapse into sleepiness during the day, or indeed, upon wakening. It seems that certain seizures are influenced by changes in an individual's level of arousal and wakefulness. Nocturnal seizures and parasomnias can sometimes be confused so it is important to be able to give a good description of what happens to the physician or even a video recording of the event if there is any doubt about the diagnosis.

## Sleep Apnoea

This is a sleep-related breathing disorder where there are regular interruptions to normal breathing. Breathing obstruction results in loud snoring, and sometimes choking noises. Typically, there are periods during which the individual stops breathing altogether, sometimes for 20 to 30 seconds, and then restarts breathing suddenly and often noisily. Sleep apnoea can significantly affect the quality of night-time sleep and is associated with excessive daytime sleepiness (Shapiro, 1993). Although not common, sleep apnoea is specifically mentioned since it often passes undetected. It is known to be more common in people with Down's Syndrome and in people who are overweight. Cases of suspected sleep apnoea should be referred to a physician who, again, will need to have a good description of what actually happens. Snoring on its own does not amount to sleep apnoea.

## Excessive Daytime Sleepiness

Any inability to sustain wakefulness must be a concern since it greatly affects quality of life. There are many reasons why an individual may be prone to fall asleep. Sometimes it is through boredom and lack of stimulation. It may also be a side effect of drugs (see chapter by Ahmed in this volume).

However, at other times there may be an untreated sleep disorder (e.g. sleep apnoea, narcolepsy, insufficient sleep). Particular attention should be paid to involuntary sleeping, that is, where a person is *unable* to remain awake. If this happens, referral should be made to a physician with a detailed description of what occurs, how often, and in what circumstances.

## Conclusion

Sleep difficulties constitute a major problem for many people. Insufficient attention has been paid to the sleep requirements and sleep problems of people with intellectual disabilities and much more research is required. However, sleep problems do occur and are commonly reported by carers as significantly affecting an individual's life and also the lives of others in the household. This chapter has attempted to provide a preliminary understanding of the sleep process and how it can become disordered. It has also made some suggestions on how to assess sleep problems and how to manage them more effectively. In such a short article it is impossible to be comprehensive and the reader is encouraged to dip into some of the publications mentioned in the reference list to obtain further information.

## References

American Sleep Disorders Association (1990) *The International Classification of Sleep Disorders; Diagnostic and Coding Manual.* Rochester, MN.: A.S.D.A.

Espie, C.A. (1991) *The Psychological Treatment of Insomnia.* Chichester and New York: J. Wiley and Sons.

Espie, C.A., Paul, A., Mcfie, J., Amos, P., Hamilton, D., Tarassenko, L., & Pardey, J. (1997) Sleep studies from a sample of adults with severe/profound mental retardation plus epilepsy. *American Journal on Mental Retardation.* (in press).

Horne, J. (1990) *Why we Sleep: The functions of sleep in humans and other mammals.* Oxford & New York : Oxford University Press.

Quine, L. (1993) Working with parents: the management of sleep disturbance in children with learning disabilities, in C. Kiernan (ed.) *Research into Practice: Implications of Research on the Challenging Behaviour of People with Learning Disabilities.* Wolverhampton: British Institute of Learning Disabilities.

Quine, L. (1997) *Solving Children's Sleep Problems: A step by step guide for parents.* Huntingdon, Cambridgeshire: Beckett-Karlson.

Simonds, J. and Parraga, H. (1982) Prevalence of sleep disorders and sleep behaviours in children and adolescents. *Journal of the American Academy of Child Psychiatry, 21, 383-388.*

Shapiro, C. (1993)  *ABC of Sleep Disorders*. London: BMJ. Publishing
    Group.

**Colin A. Espie**  is Professor of Clinical Psychology and Head of
    Department of Psychological Medicine at the University of Glasgow.
    Prior to this appointment he was clinical director of learning disability
    services in Ayrshire, Scotland.  Professor Espie has conducted numerous
    research studies on sleep disorders and on epilepsy.  He has published
    widely in these areas.

**Contact Address**
    University of Glasgow,
    Department of Psychological Medicine
    Academic Centre
    Gartnavel Royal Hospital
    GLASGOW G12 0XH.
    Scotland.

# 9

# *Reducing Antipsychotic Drugs*

## Zamir Ahmed

In the field of intellectual disability the use of antipsychotic drugs is widespread. They are used to alleviate the symptoms of mental illness but their greater use is in modification of problematic behaviour. Much controversy surrounds the latter use. The prevailing opinion is to minimise their use and if they are already prescribed, attempt to taper them off.

The problems with antipsychotic drugs is the side effects associated with their use, especially the long term side effects.

This chapter will look at the effectiveness of antipsychotic drugs in modifying behaviour; the problems associated with antipsychotic drugs; the difficulties encountered with drug reduction and offer some points to consider when reducing antipsychotic drugs.

### *Prevalence Of Antipsychotic Drug Use*

Large numbers of people with intellectual difficulties are on antipsychotic medication. Most surveys, which have measured the prevalence of antipsychotic drug use, show that for a hospital population the range is between 22% and 45% of individuals where as for those living in the community the figure clusters around 20%. It has also been shown that 9% - 26%, of those taking antipsychotic drugs, are on more than one type of antipsychotic drug.

The commonest antipsychotic drugs used in the treatment of behavioural problems are: thioridazine, chlorpromazine and haloperidol. Looking at the prevalence of mental illness; which is the main indication for prescribing antipsychotic drugs (including personality disorder), it ranges between 8-15% and those with a psychotic illness constitute 4-6% (Deb & Fraser (1994)). Thus the use of antipsychotic drugs is much greater than the prevalence of mental illness especially psychotic illness in this population. This would suggest that the discrepancy is due to the use of these drugs for behavioural problems.

Aggressive behaviour is the strongest predictor of antipsychotic drug use but other behaviours include self injurious behaviour, self stimulation (stereotypy) and tantrums.

Within institutional setting, those individuals who are violent and destructive, and have high levels of physical skills, motor skills and self direction are the ones most likely to receive antipsychotic drugs. Other factors are also important in determining if an individual is placed on antipsychotic drugs for a behavioural problem; such as staff perception of the behaviour, environmental factors, staff ratio and administrative treatment philosophies.

## *Effectiveness Of Antipsychotic Drugs*

The useful of antipsychotic drugs at controlling problematic behaviour remains debatable. There have been numerous published studies which have favoured the use of these drugs for behavioural problems, however, reviews by Sprague & Werry, (1971) and Aman & Singh (1988) showed that the vast majority of these studies were methodologically flawed and thus inconclusive. However both reviews noted that antipsychotic drugs may be useful in controlling *some* behaviors in *some* people.

Recent, methodologically more sound studies, have shown some benefit. For example, Singh & Aman (1981) showed thioridazine to be helpful in reducing hyperactivity, bizarre behaviour and stereotypy. Aman White & Field (1984) showed a reduction in stereotypy with chlorpromazine. Gualteiri & Schroeder (1989) treated 15 adults with severe intellectual disability with fluphenazine in an open and double blind design and found a 30% reduction in self injurious behaviour over a six month period. Singh & Qwino (1992) in an open and double blind study reported improvement in behaviour in 52 individuals with zuclopenthixol compared with placebo. These findings for the usefulness of zuclopenthixol have also been reported by Izmeth Khan Kumarajuewa Shivanathan, Veall, & Wiley (1988). Vanden Borre, Vermote, Butiëns, Thiry, Dierick, Geutjens, Sieben, & Heylen, (1993) in a double blind placebo controlled cross-over add-on therapy with risperidone, reported it to be better than a placebo at controlling problem behaviour, which was measured using the Aberrant Behaviour Checklist and Global Clinical Impression Scale. Campbell & Spencer (1988) reported haloperidol to significantly reduce stereotypic behaviour in a sample of children with autism.

From the various studies the evidence for use of antipsychotic drugs in managing behavioural problems is strongest for control of stereotypy. This is further reinforced by animal studies, which show that antipsychotic drugs counteract stimulant drug induced stereotypy in rats (Aman, 1982).

## Problems with Antipsychotic Drugs

Although antipsychotic drugs are useful in the treatment of mental illness and play a role in management of behavioural problems, they are not without their difficulties. They have both short term side effects, which occur soon after starting the drug and long term side effects, which become evident after prolonged use.

The short term side effects are many and varied. Once they occur they can follow a number of courses: they may diminish with time, they may be controlled by other drugs, the individual may develop tolerance to the side effects or they will to go away once the drug is stopped. Antipsychotic drugs effect many organs of the body including the brain, through their action on various neurotransmitter systems.

Mental illness occurs through their ability to block the action of Dopamine. This is one of the many neurotransmitters found in the brain, which transmits messages between nerve cells. It is this blockade of the dopamine receptors in the mesolimbic region of the brain that is responsible for the antipsychotic effect and it is blockade of dopamine at other receptor sites which is responsible for the side effects. For example, dopamine receptor blockade in the extrapyramidal system, which is involved with control of movement, is responsible for majority of the side effects of antipsychotic drugs. These can be divided into four types, which are collectively known as extrapyramidal side effects.

### Extrapyramidal Side Effects.

**1. Pseudo-Parkinsonism** leads to symptoms which are similar to those encountered in Parkinson's disease namely, stiffness, loss of facial expression, tremor and a shuffling gait.

**2. Acute dystonias** are painful muscle spasms often affecting the neck or the eyes and require emergency treatment to alleviate.

**3. Akathesia** is probably the most common side effect associated with antipsychotic drugs and can occur in up to 50% of cases. It is characterised by the individual feeling restless or agitated. This is accompanied by increased activity such as foot tapping, rocking or pacing. Akathesia is not a pleasant experience and in a person with an intellectual disability who may not be able to communicate their distress the outward signs may be mistaken for worsening of their behavioural disorder.

Except for tardive dyskinesia (see below) these side effects tend to develop in the first three months and they can be ameliorated by use of anticholinergic or other drugs.

**4. Tardive dyskinesia** is usually a late onset side effect of antipsychotic drugs which develops after few years of treatment but can develop much sooner. Tardive dyskinesia is defined as: late onset involuntary (not under conscious control), irregular, choreoathetoid (jerky and purposeless) movements of the head, trunk and limbs; first described by Schonecker in 1957. These movements commonly affect the mouth region leading to darting, protruding and twisting movements of the tongue. They can be minimal, hardly noticed or maximal and they are cosmetically and physically incapacitating.

The reported prevalence of tardive dyskinesia in people with intellectual disability varies between 30-45%. This variation is probably due to differences in defining and rating tardive dyskinesia rather than a true difference in prevalence. It has also been noted that those with mental illness and intellectual disability are at a greater risk of tardive dyskinesia. Cohen, Khan, Zheng, & Chiles (1991) found a prevalence of 47% in those that had schizophrenia compared with 17% who did not have a psychotic illness.

Although Antipsychotic drugs can produce tardive dyskinesia, in the early stages they also mask the symptoms of tardive dyskinesia such that when they are withdrawn the tardive dyskinesia becomes evident.

Once the tardive dyskinesia develops, then in approximately 50% of cases it is irreversible, even if antipsychotic drugs are stopped. Thus it can have very serious implications as it is cosmetically disfiguring and causes physical morbidity. In severe cases it can effect the muscles of respiration and very occasionally it can be fatal.

Other factors are also associated with the risk of developing tardive dyskinesia. The risk increases with duration of antipsychotic drugs (Kane, & Smith, 1982), co-prescription of anticholinergic drugs (Gardos, & Cole, (1983), Gualteiri, Schroeder, Hicks, & Quade, 1986), presence of affective disorder (Davis, Berger & Hollister, 1976; Mukherjee, Rosen, Caracci, 1986), pervious extrapyramidal side effects (Jeste, Potkins, Sinha, Feder, & Wyatt, 1979), increasing age, in females and in those that have diffuse brain pathology (Kane & Smith, 1982). Although various strategies have been tried in order to treat tardive dyskinesia none have been truly successful (Goetz & Kiawans, 1984).

Tardive dyskinesia is a common long term sequelae of antipsychotic drug use, it is a serious problem causing much suffering and in about half of the cases it is irreversible. To date there is no cure for it and people with intellectual disabilities, who have increased risk of having diffuse cerebral damage, are at a greater risk of developing tardive dyskinesia. Due to the potential irreversibility of tardive dyskinesia and also the problems surrounding valid consent from people with an intellectual disability, the use of antipsychotic drugs presents doctors with serious medico-legal implications.

### Prolactin Effects

The release of the hormone prolactin from the pituitary gland is controlled by dopamine, dopamine cuts down the amount of prolactin released by the pituitary gland. Antipsychotic drugs by blocking the action of dopamine increase the release of prolactin from the pituitary gland. The increase in the level of prolactin can lead to breast enlargement, production of breast milk, impotence in males, amenorrhoea and can lead to a false pregnancy test.

### Anticholinergic Effects

These occur when antipsychotic drugs block the action of the neurotransmitter, acetylcholine, within the brain or other parts of the body. Within the brain the main effect is to cause delirium, this is quite rare and effects mostly the elderly. The peripheral antichloinergic side effects include blurred vision, dry mouth, fast heart rate, constipation, impotence in males, and problems passing urine.

### Other Side Effects

These include effects on the skin, leading to skin rashes and increased sensitivity to sunlight, making the person more prone to sunburns and necessitating the use of sun block creams. Antipsychotic drugs can also cause increased pigmentation of the skin such that the person becomes darker in color.

Antipsychotic drugs especially thioridazine in very high doses can effect the eyes leading to a condition called retinitis pigmentosa which can lead to blindness.

Effects on the heart can lead to arrhythmia's and also changes in the electrocardiogram (ECG), these can be fatal. They can also cause a drop in the white cell count in the blood, leading to an increased risk of infection.

Also the threshold for seizures can be lowered and this makes a person with epilepsy more prone to suffer seizures, which is an important consideration in intellectually disabled population where about 30% also suffer with epilepsy.

A common side effect is a drop in blood pressure when a person rises to a standing position, this can cause dizziness or can cause a person to pass out and thus there is a risk of injury. Luckily tolerance develops rapidly to this side effect. Sedation and weight gain are also very common.

Effects on the liver can lead to jaundice.

A more serious but rare complication of antipsychotic drugs is a disorder called neuroleptic malignant syndrome. The individual develops a fever, becomes very stiff, level of consciousness fluctuates, blood pressure and heart rate tend to go up and down. There is an increase in the level of an enzyme called creatinine phosphokinase detected in the blood. This condition requires the antipsychotic drug be immediate stopped and intensive medical care. It carries a death rate of around 10%.

## The Decline In Use Of Antipsychotic Drugs

The publication by Lipman (1970), which showed that there was a high use of antipsychotic drugs in people with learning disabilities, and a review by Sprague & Werry (1971) highlighting methodological flaws in those studies which showed a positive outcome in treatment of problematic behaviours, gave ground for debating the usefulness of antipsychotic drugs in treating behavioural problems. However, it was the involvement of the legal system, in the USA, in the case of Wyatt v Stickney (1972), that had a more marked influence on the use of antipsychotic drugs in clinical practice and led to efforts to decrease their use. It also led to establishment of guidelines for use of antipsychotic drugs (Rinck, Guidry & Calkins, 1989). The case of Garrity v Gallen USA (1981) (Rinck, Guidry & Calkins 1989)) added three other conditions (see Box).

There were also a number of Court cases in which individuals were awarded damages as a result of suffering harm from the inappropriate use of antipsychotic drugs. The first of these, which was a milestone and responsible for opening the floodgate for other such cases, was Clites v State of Iowa USA (1982) (Rinck, Guidry & Calkins (1989)). It was the first case in which the development of tardive dyskinesia as a result of antipsychotic drug use was taken to Court. Clites was a 17 year old male with a intellectual disability who had been treated with thioridazine for sexual misconduct and aggression, by a consultant psychiatrist. The primary physician further increased the dose and added other antipsychotic drugs. There was no further contact from a psychiatrist for 5 years, a physical examination was not performed for 2½ years. The antipsychotic drugs were continued despite deterioration in a fairly high functioning individual and the development of tardive dyskinesia. Clites was awarded $760,165 as compensation.

---

### Guidelines for the use of antipsychotic drugs

1. Medication to be given only after written orders from a physician.
2. Written records of medication to be kept with each persons chart.
3. Weekly review of drugs.
4. Termination date not to exceed 30 days.
5. Patients to be free of any unnecessary or excessive drugs.
6. Written notes to be kept on the effects of psycho-active drugs.
7. Medication not to be used as punishment, convenience or as a substitute for rehabilitation programme.
8. Trained pharmacist to review drug charts.
9. Trained staff to administer drugs.
10. Psychotropic drugs only to be given based on documented individual needs.
11. To be given as part of an overall comprehensive individual plan.
12. Each person should be evaluated for possible dosage reduction.

---

Following this case, malpractice suits increased on behalf of persons developing tardive dyskinesia; for example, in Falgenbaum v Oakland Medical Centre USA (1986), the plaintiff was awarded $378,000 which was recovered from private citizens; the physicians and drug companies. In Heidin v USA (1985), Heidin was a Vietnam veteran, he was prescribed antipsychotic drugs after he admitted himself for alcohol detoxification, following 5 years of antipsychotic drug treatment he developed severe tardive dyskinesia. The courts awarded him more than $2 million.

The guidelines and awards for tardive dyskinesia issued by the legal system, forced States in the USA to rationalise and minimise the use of antipsychotic drugs especially for behavioural problems. The negative image of antipsychotic medication was further tainted by research carried out by Dr. Stephen E Breuning at the Coldwater Regional Centre for Developmental Disabilities in Michigan USA. His research showed that antipsychotic drugs had a negative impact on learning ability and that at low doses they were no better at controlling behavior than placebo and at high doses actually made the behaviour worse. These studies had a major impact in the field of learning disability, although it was later discovered that these studies by Dr. Breuning had apparently been fabricated (Aman & Singh, 1986).

By late 1980s, 90% of the states in America had regulations regarding use of antipsychotic drugs (Rinck, Guidry & Calkins, 1989). This led to increased scrutiny of the use of antipsychotic drugs especially through the involvement of inter-disciplinary teams (Briggs, 1989), the use of behavioural data to determine effectiveness of antipsychotic drugs (Glaser & Morreau, 1986) and the review of drug charts by clinical pharmacist (Inoue, 1982).

The prescription of antipsychotic drugs was reduced as a consequence of guidelines introduced by the courts. Mendola, Zaharia & Carver (1980), reported a reduction from 27% to 20% usage over a 3½ year period following quarterly reviews. They also stated that many individuals had been taken off antipsychotics completely; with positive results, e.g. improved skill building, or at least with no deterioration of their behaviour. White (1983) showed a decrease from 26.4% to 14.5% in use of antipsychotic drugs. Schalock, Harper & Genung (1981) reported a decline from 30.5% usage in 1981 to 20% by 1983. Poindexter (1989) showed a decrease from 33.3% to 9.5% over a 10 year period, although in this study it was noted that the average daily dose actually increased. Briggs (1989) noted a decline in antipsychotic usage over a 4 year period with the rate stabilizing around 14%.

These studies clearly showed that reduction in antipsychotic drug use was possible. However it also became evident that some individuals did not fair too well after drug reduction and the antipsychotic drug had to be re-instated. Research needed to focus on what factors influenced drug reduction such that if these could be controlled, the individual then would have the best chance of coming off antipsychotic drugs.

## *Factors Influencing Drug Reduction*

There are not many studies which have systematically looked at factors which influence antipsychotic drug reduction in people with intellectual disabilities in whom the drug has been used to control a behavioural problem. However three studies will be discussed.

### Chadsey-Rusch and Sprague (1989)

This was a hospital based study looking at factors distinguishing successful and unsuccessful drug reduction in 105 individuals in which 84 had their antipsychotic medication dose reduced by a third every three months while the other 21 individuals used as a control group. Changes in behaviour were monitored by looking at accounts of the behaviour recorded by staff in the case notes. Of the people who underwent a drug reduction 25% were drug free at end of the study, 75% went back onto their antipsychotic medication. When they looked at difference between those that had come off the medication and those that went back on, they found the following:

1. The 'drug re-instated' group differed most on disruptive behaviour, self stimulation and physical aggression compared to the 'drug free' group.
2. They also noted that maladaptive behaviour in the re-instated group was worse when drug dosage had reached a minimal level. This was also the case for positive and neutral behaviours, which suggested that antipsychotic drugs may also be suppressing these more desirable behaviours.
3. They found that the frequency of maladaptive behavior did not differ between the re-instated, drug free and control groups and thus questioned the reason for reinstating the drug. However, they did not take into account the severity or intensity of the behaviour.
4. They also stated that staff perception of maladaptive behaviour in combination with favourable attitudes toward drug treatment, influenced the decision to maintain residents on antipsychotic drugs more than objective counts of target behaviour.

### Luchins, Dojka & Hanrahan (1993)

This was a retrospective study looking at the clinical notes of 95 individuals from one unit for a 3 month period in 1984 and again for a 3 month period in 1989. Individuals with and without a mental illness were included in the study. All the individuals in this unit had a review of their antipsychotic medication every 6 months and attempts were made to reduce the medication at each review. In the 5 year period between 1984 and 1989 some people were completely off their medication whereas in others antipsychotic medication had to be re-instated. Looking at the difference between these two groups they found that:

1. the presence of psychosis was significantly associated with reinstatement of antipsychotic drug.

2. Alternative drugs to control behaviors such as lithium, propranolol, buspirone and carbamazepine were associated with a reduction in antipsychotic drug usage of both those with or without a psychotic illness.
3. Age, gender, initial level of learning disability or behaviour severity did not effect the outcome.
4. Taken overall, a reduction in dosage of drug was found to be associated with improvement, rather than a deterioration in behaviour.

## Branford (1996)

The most recent study is by Branford (1996) carried out in Leicestershire, UK. The previous two studies only looked at individuals in a hospital setting whereas this study addressed both hospital and community populations. In this study 123 patients were included; living in hospitals or supported community accommodation. Drugs were reduced on a monthly basis with an aim to reduce by one third of original dose each month but this varied and in some cases the reduction period extended over 8 months. The study lasted for 12 months in total. Prior to drug reduction, demographic data was obtained via case notes and structured interviews with carers. Behaviour level was rated using the Aberrant Behaviour Checklist (ABC) and the Reiss Screen for Maladaptive Behaviour. Psychiatric status was measured using the psychopathology inventory for mentally retarded adults (PIMRA). At end of the study the individuals were divided into 3 groups; group 1, (25%), consisted of individuals who were drug free at the end of the study period; group 2, (42%), in whom drug reduction had to be stopped or drugs re-instated because of deterioration in behaviour, and group 3, (33%), who neither completed the drug reduction or experienced any deterioration in behaviour.

Comparing group 1, the 'drug free' group and group 2, the drug 're-instated' group, the following was noted:
1. There was no difference between the drug free group or the drug re-instated group for sex, degree of learning disability or the concurrent use of lithium, carbamazepine or antichloinergic drugs,.
2. Successful withdrawal was associated with:-
   a) Presence of epilepsy
   b) Low initial Chlorpromazine equivalent dose of less than 100 mg.
   c) Prescription of thioridazine.
   d) Lower PIMRA Scores for schizophrenia and Affective Disorder.
   e) Lower Reiss Scores for aggression, autism, self injury and overactivity.

f) Lower ABC Scores for stereotypy, hyperactivity and irritability.
g) Lower level of ability to understand instructions.
h) Poor hearing.

In summary these studies suggested that people with a mental illness tended to need to continue antipsychotic drugs. A person's age, sex and level of disability were not associated with outcome of drug reduction; behaviour tended to be worse at minimal doses; use of alternative drugs may be of some benefit and most importantly the attitudes of care givers towards drug reduction and the individuals behaviour were very important in determining outcome.

## Problems With Antipsychotic Drug Reduction

The use of 'drug holidays', was initially recommended for individuals on antipsychotic drugs as it was felt that if a person was free from antipsychotic drugs for a short period and then restarted this would decrease the risk of tardive dyskinesia. However, this proved to be a false assumption and many reports showed that drug holidays were in fact associated with increased risk of developing irreversible tardive dyskinesia; Branchey & Branchey (1984).

It also became evident that some people with intellectual disability show a deterioration in behaviour as a consequence of attempts to withdraw them from antipsychotic drugs. Zimmerman & Heistad (1982) noted that in 40% of subjects in their study who had a reduction of antipsychotic drug, there was a marked deterioration in self stimulation, self abuse, verbal and physical aggression and shouting. Briggs (1989) showed that 33% of patients had their antipsychotic drugs re-instated after attempts at drug reduction. Fielding, Murphy, Reagan & Peterson (1980) showed that those who had unsuccessful drug reduction had a significant increase in maladaptive behaviour compared to baseline behaviour. Gualteiri, Schroeder, Hicks & Quade (1986) also noted that antipsychotic drug withdrawal may lead to a non-dyskinetic withdrawal syndrome which consists of nausea, vomiting, anorexia and weight loss.

In about 24% of individuals behaviour may get worse, with hyperactivity, aggression, agitation, destructiveness mood changes, and tantrums. This behaviour tends to be different from the original behaviour problem and usually lasts for about 4 months (Kalachnik (1996))

As stated previously antipsychotic drugs mask early signs of tardive dyskinesia, so any attempt to withdraw them can lead to emergent tardive dyskinesia. In fact emergent tardive dyskinesia can be expected in up to 67% of cases. Of those in whom tardive dyskinesia is uncovered, it will dissipate in about 50% of cases usually within 3-4 months. Although the high rate of emergent tardive dyskinesia may sound alarming, it is important to remember that the earlier one detects tardive dyskinesia and stops antipsychotic drugs the greater chance that it will be reversible for a given individual.

## Guidelines For Drug Reduction

This section applies to people with an intellectual disability who do not have a psychotic illness and in whom antipsychotic medication is used to control problem behaviour. If a decision is made to use antipsychotic drugs to control a problem behaviour, it is important to quantify the behaviour by measuring its frequency, duration, severity and impact on the environment including other people. Once the drug is started then regular review of the behaviour is needed to establish whether a drug is working and how well it is working. It is important to review the antipsychotic medication on a regular basis to see if it needs to be continued.

The following points need to be considered if deciding to reduce and stop an antipsychotic drug:

1. A decision to withdraw the antipsychotic drug has to be made on a multidisciplinary level, addressing staff anxieties about drug withdrawal.
2. It is very important to educate all the team members about why drug withdrawal is being attempted and the dangers of continued drug use. Any anxieties or disagreements at the multidisciplinary level can easily jeopardise attempts at drug withdrawal.
3. The next stage is to record what the individual's baseline behaviour is like prior to drug reduction, this should preferably be done for a period of about 1 month, noting fluctuations in the level of behaviour and those events which exacerbate the behaviour. This will give an idea of the background fluctuation in the behaviour such that if this occurs during the drug reduction it is not attributed to the process of drug reduction.
4. It needs to be decided what measures will be taken if there is any deterioration in behaviour during drug reduction, these may include use of alternative drugs, recruiting a greater number of staff for a short period or involving the help of an intensive support team.
5. The drug reduction itself can range from 25% reduction in dose every month to 10% reduction in dose every 3 months.

6. Behaviour should be assessed regularly, remembering that in about a quarter of cases there will be an acute deterioration in behaviour which can last about 4 months.
7. Also emergent tardive dyskinesia has to be anticipated in over 50% of cases and its form and severity recorded.

# References

Aman, M.G. (1982) Stimulant drug effects in developmental disorders and hyperactivity: toward resolution of disparate findings. *Journal of Autism and Developmental Disorders*, 12, 385-395.

Aman & Singh (1986) A critical appraisal of recent drug research in mental retardation: The Coldwater Studies. *Journal of Mental Deficiency Research*, 30, 203-216

Aman & Singh (1988) Patterns of drug use, methodological considerations, measurement techniques and future trends. In: *Psychopharmacology of Developmental Disabilities*. New York; Springer Verlag.

Aman, M.G., Field, C.J., Bridgeman, G. (1985). City wide survey of drug patterns amongst non-institutionalised mentally retarded persons. *Applied research in Mental Retardation*, 6, 159-171.

Aman, M.G., White, A.J., & Field C.J. (1984). Chlorpromazine effects on stereotypic and conditioned behaviour of severely retarded patients - a pilot study. *Journal of Mental Deficiency Research*, 28, 253-260.

Branchey, M. & Branchey L. (1984) Patterns of psychotropic drug use and tardive dyskinesia. *Journal of Clinical Psychopharmacology*, 4, 41-45

Branford, D. (1996) Factors associated with the successful or unsuccessful withdrawal of antipsychotic drug therapy prescribed for people with learning disabilities. *Journal of Intellectual Disability Research*, 40, 4, 322-329.

Briggs (1989). Monitoring and evaluating psychotropic drug use for persons with mental retardation: A follow up report. *American Journal on Mental Retardation*, 93, 633-639.

Campbell, M. & Spencer, E.K. (1988) Psychopharmacology in child and adolescent psychiatry: a review of the past five years. *Journal of the American Academy of Child and Adolescent Psychiatry*, 27, 269-279.

Chadsey-Rusch, J., & Sprague, R.L. (1989). Maladaptive Behaviours associated with neuroleptic drug maintenance. *American Journal on Mental Retardation*, 93, 607-617.

Cohen, S., Khan, A., Zheng, Y. & Chiles, J. (1991) Tardive dyskinesia in the mentally retarded: comparison of prevalence, risk factors, and topography with a schizophrenic population. *Acta Psychiatrica Scandinavica,* 83, 234-237.

Davis, K., Berger, P., & Hollister, L. (1976). Tardive dyskinesia and depressive illness. *Psychopharmacology*, 2, 125.

Deb, S. & Fraser, W.I (1994) The Use of Psychotropic Medication in People with Learning Disability: Towards Rational Prescribing. *Human Psychopharmacology*, 9, 259-272.

Fielding, L.T., Murphy, R.J., Reagan, M.W., & Peterson, J.L. (1980). An assessment programme to reduce drug use with the mentally retarded. *Hospital and Community Psychiatry*, 31, 11, 771-773.

Gardos, G., & Cole, J.O. (1983). Tardive dyskinesia and anticholinergic drugs. *American Journal of Psychiatry*, 140, 200-2.

Glaser, B. A., & Morreau, L. E. (1986) Effects of interdisciplinary team review on the use of antipsychotic agents with severely and profoundly mentally handicapped persons. *American Journal of Mental Deficiency*, 90, 371-9.

Goetz, C.G., Kiawans, H.L. (1984). Tardive dyskinesia. *Neurologic Clinics*, 2.

Gualteiri, C.T. & Schroeder, S.R. (1989) Pharmacotherapy for self-injurious behaviour: preliminary tests of the D1 hypothesis. Psychopharmacology Bulletin, 25, 364-371.

Gualteiri, C.T., Schroeder, S.R., Hicks, R.E., & Quade, D. (1986). Tardive dyskinesia in young mentally retarded individuals. *Archives of General Psychiatry*, 43, 335-340.

Inoue, F. (1982). A clinical pharmacy service to reduce psychotropic medication use in an institution for mentally handicapped persons. *Mental Retardation*, 20, 70-74.

Izmeth, M.G., Khan, S.Y., Kumarajuewa, D.I., Shivanathan, S., Veall, R.M., & Wiley, Y.V. (1988). Zuclopenthixol decanoate in the management of behavioural disorders in mentally handicapped patients. *Pharmatherapeutica*, 5, 4, 217-227.

Jeste, D.V., Potkins, S. G., Sinha, S., Feder, S., & Wyatt, R.J. (1979) Tardive Dyskinesia: Reversible and Persistent. *Archives of General Psychiatry*, 36, 585-594

Kalachnik, J.E. (1996) Lowest "optimal effective dose" (OED). Rational Approaches to Psychotropic Medications Seminar presented at Woodward, IA.

Kane & Smith (1982). Tardive dyskinesia: prevalence and risk factors *Archives of General Psychiatry*, 39, 473-81.

La Mendola, W., Zaharia, E., & Carver, M. (1980). Reducing psychotropic drug use in an institution for the retarded. *Hospital and Community Psychiatry*, 31, 271-272.

Lipman, R.S. (1970). The use of psychopharmacological agents in residential facilities for the retarded. In F.J. Menolascino (ed.) *Psychiatric Approaches to Mental Retardation*. New York: Basic Books.

Luchins, D. J., Dojka, D. & Hanrahan , P. (1993). Factors associated with reduction in antipsychotic medication dosage in adults with mental retardation. *American Journal on Mental Retardation*, 98, 1, 165-175.

Mukherjee, S., Rosen, A., M., Caracci, G. (1986). Persistent tardive dyskinesia in bipolar patients. *Archives of General Psychiatry*, 43, 342-6.

Poindexter, A.R. (1989). Psychotropic drug patterns in a large ICF/MR facility. A ten-year experience. *American Journal on Mental Retardation*, 93, 6, 624-26.

Rinck, Guidry & Calkins (1989). Review of States' practices on the use of psychotropic medication'. *American Journal on Mental Retardation*, 93, 6, 657-668.

Schalock, R., Harper, R.S. & Genung, T. (1981). Community integration of mentally retarded adults. *American Journal of Mental Deficiency*, 85, 478-488.

Singh, I. & Qwino, W.J.E. (1992) A double blind comparison of zuclopenthixol tablets with placebo in the treatment of mentally handicapped in-patients with associated behavioural disorders. *Journal of Intellectual Disability Research*, 36, 6, 541-550.

Singh, N. N., & Aman, M.G. (1981). Effects of thioridazine dosage on the behaviour of severely mentally retarded persons. *American Journal of Mental Deficiency*, 85, 580-7.

Sprague, R.L., & Werry, J (1971). Methodology of psychopharmacological studies with the retarded. In N.R. Ellis (ed.) *International Review of Research into Mental Retardation (Vol 5)*. New York: Academic Press.

Vanden Borre, R. Vermote, R. Butiëns, M. Thiry, P. Dierick, P.J. Geutjens, J. Sieben, G. & Heylen, S. (1993). Risperidone as add-on therapy in behavioural disturbances in mental retardation: a double-blind placebo-controlled cross-over study. *Acta Psychiatrica Scandinavica*, 87, 167-171

White, A. (1983). Changing patterns of psychoactive drug use with the mentally retarded. *New Zealand Medical Journal*, 96, 686-8

Zimmerman, R.L. & Heistad, G.T.,. (1982). Studies of the long-term efficacy of antipsychotic drugs in controlling the behaviour of institutionalized retardates. *Journal of the American Academy of Child Psychiatry.* 21, 136-143.

**Zamir Ahmed** qualified at the University of Wales, College of Medicine. Initially he pursued a career in general medicine before embarking on psychiatry. He currently works as a lecturer in psychological medicine at the University of Wales, College of Medicine. His research interests focus on psychopharmacology in the field of learning disabilities and the genetics of epilepsy.

**Contact Address**
Welsh Centre for Learning Disability
Meridian Court
North Road
Cardiff CF4 3BL
Wales

# 10
## *New Advances in the Treatment of Epilepsy: Do New Drugs Mean New Hope?*

### Sheila Wallace

Antiepileptic drugs (AEDs) are the main approach to the treatment of epilepsy. The answer to the question, "do new drugs mean new hope?" is undoubtedly "yes", but a knowledge of the drugs themselves, the circumstances in which each of the new drugs is most likely to be helpful and of the possible adverse effects are equally essential, if the best results are to be obtained.

Vigabatrin, lamotrigine and gabapentin are those new drugs for which there is the most available information, but early reports on tiagabine and topiramate are now appearing. When using drugs, and any other form of treatment for epilepsy, it is important to consider the aims. Improvement in seizure control is undoubtedly the main objective. However, better seizure control should not be attained at the expense of side effects. Thus, the presence of over-sedation, proven specific adverse effects on learning ability, or general physical illness should make the physician re-assess the usefulness of the new drug. Some of the newer AEDs can precipitate psychiatric disturbances.

It is essential to appreciate that a learning-disabled person might not be able to describe adverse effects, particularly if these cause alterations in thought processes, depression or mood changes. Seizure control can even, in some circumstances, make the person with learning difficulties more difficult to look after: this occurs particularly when non-convulsive status epilepticus is controlled and the learning-disabled person becomes more alert and active. Although increase in independence must always be a goal, the quality of life of the carer should not be completely ignored.

This chapter looks at the characteristics of four new drugs; lamotrigine, vigabatrin, gabapentin and topiramate with brief reference to three others; oxcarbazepine, felbamate and tiagabine, in relation to their efficacy, safety, effects on behaviour and cognition and either reported, or estimated, quality of life.

## Lamotrigine

Lamotrigine is dispensed in either solid tablets or tablets which are chewable and which disperse when added to water. The latter formulation has a blackcurrant flavour and seems acceptable to young children and others who cannot swallow solid tablets.

### Treatment Spectrum

Lamotrigine has a wide antiepileptic spectrum (Brodie 1992; Besag, Wallace, Dulac, Alving, Spencer & Hosking, 1995; Wallace, 1994). The initial trials in human subjects were done on adults with partial seizures, but widening of the range of seizures and epilepsies for which lamotrigine was given soon led to the realisation that lamotrigine could be very effective in the control of seizures which do not respond readily to the more established AEDs, eg phenobarbitone, phenytoin, carbamazepine and valproate. It is useful to consider specifically the seizures and epilepsies for which lamotrigine should be considered an early choice, giving particular attention to severe epilepsies which occur almost exclusively in learning disabled children or adults.

**West syndrome** is characterised by the onset, in the first year of life, of infantile spasms. In a spasm the baby suddenly throws the arms out to the side, draws the knees up and may let out a scream. (It is easy to confuse infantile spasms with colic). The electroencephalogram (EEG) shows a very characteristic severe abnormality, hypsarrhythmia. The baby either loses the ability to perform skills which have been learned or fails to learn any new skills. Surveys of children who had had West syndrome about 30 years ago found that at least 85 per cent of them later had severe intellectual disabilities, and a further 10 per cent had some problems in school and with their behaviour. There is some evidence to suggest that if the spasms are controlled soon after they begin the intellectual outlook is better. Lamotrigine has been used successfully for a small proportion of children with West syndrome who have failed to respond to other AED (Schlumberger, Chavez, Palacios, Rey, Pajot & Dulac, 1994). It would be difficult to suggest that lamotrigine should be the first choice AED for West syndrome, since it must be introduced slowly, and the maximum maintenance dose may be reached only after two to three months. Nevertheless, lamotrigine can be effective when other AED have failed.

The **Lennox Gastaut** syndrome is characterised by onset in the second or third years of life of a mixed seizure disorder, with tonic seizures and atypical absences predominating. Epileptic drop attacks, which are usually tonic, but can be atonic, are the most physically disabling aspect of this syndrome. Intellectual difficulties are always present. In the early studies of patients, particularly children, with mixed seizure disorders, it became apparent that lamotrigine could be very effective in the control of the epileptic drop attacks, thus leading to overall improvement in the physical status of affected patients (Wallace, 1989; Schlumberger, Chavez, Palacios, Rey, Pajot & Dulac, 1994). The early data was followed by specific studies in both adults and children which showed that lamotrigine could definitely improve seizure control in the Lennox Gastaut syndrome (Timmings & Richens, 1992; Oller, Russi & Oller Daurella 1991). More recently, a double-blind placebo-controlled trial of lamotrigine, when used as add-on therapy to other AED, has shown that lamotrigine can significantly reduce the total seizure frequency, and also the frequencies of all drop attacks and of tonic-clonic seizures when these were assessed separately (Billard, Motte, Arvidsson, Trevathan, Calladai, Campos & Douglas, 1996). Clearly lamotrigine is likely to be used much earlier than previously in this condition, with hopes that the longer term outlook could improve.

In *myoclonic-astatic epilepsy*, both sudden myoclonic jerks and sudden drop attacks occur. Absence seizures can also be a feature. Learning difficulties are common, but may be absent. The role of lamotrigine in myoclonic-astatic epilepsy is not clear-cut. There is no report of worsening of the seizures when lamotrigine is given. The majority of patients have fewer atonic (drop) attacks, with the response being dramatic in some cases (Wallace 1993; Gusev, Petroukhin, Bourd, Medvedev & Mukhin, 1996). There is some anecdotal evidence that a combination of lamotrigine with valproate is more effective than either drug alone, in the treatment of myoclonic astatic epilepsy.

*Atypical absences*, regardless of accompanying seizures and of the epilepsy syndrome of which they are a component are likely to decrease in frequency by at least 50 per cent in about 50 per cent of patients treated (Besag, Wallace, Dulac, Alving, Spencer & Hosking, 1995). Reduction in absences leads to an increase in continued alertness, and helps concentration. Thus lamotrigine can make the intellectually disabled more in contact with their surroundings and more able to complete day-to-day tasks.

The numbers suffering from some of the *rarer epileptic syndromes* are very small, and it is difficult to draw more than tentative conclusions from the data available. In a small group of infants studied personally, lamotrigine has been effective in the control of the seizures in early infantile epileptic encephalopathy. Lamotrigine, combined with valproate, gives good, but not complete control in epilepsy with myoclonic absences (Manonmani & Wallace 1994). Use of the St Piers Lingfield monolog, which counts spikes, i.e. epileptic discharges, on the EEG over many hours, has demonstrated that lamotrigine can reduce epileptic discharges which may occur between obvious seizures (Besag, 1992). Lamotrigine can be very helpful in the myoclonia associated with infantile neuronal ceroid lipofuscinosis (Santavouri, Himberg, Ahola, Hosking & Yuen, 1995).

In partial seizures, lamotrigine has a proven role. A monotherapy comparison between carbamazepine and lamotrigine in adults demonstrated equal efficacy, but with fewer side effects associated with lamotrigine (Brodie, Richens & Yuen, 1995). This report referred to a trial conducted in adults with newly diagnosed epilepsy and thus the patients may not have had the same sort of brain disorders as those with chronic long-standing epilepsy and intellectual disabilities. However, when the responses to lamotrigine in children, overall, were compared with those with learning difficulties, no differences were apparent (Besag, Wallace, Dulac, Alving, Spencer & Hosking, 1995).

Lamotrigine can be used as first choice monotherapy for other seizure types, though it currently does not hold a licence for this use. In particular, lamotrigine can be very effective for drop attacks and atypical absences when used as the only medication. It is however, not yet clear how lamotrigine compares with other medications which might be used in these circumstances.

## How To Use Lamotrigine

Lamotrigine should always be introduced gradually. The recommended starting doses take concomitant AEDs into account. In particular, since valproate inhibits the metabolism of lamotrigine, a very small initial dose and very slow escalation of lamotrigine dosage are essential if a rash is to be avoided. The rash is measles-like and is most likely to occur within two to three weeks of starting lamotrigine. Should it occur, the lamotrigine must be stopped immediately. The recommended dosages for children who are on valproate are lamotrigine 0.2mg/kg/day for two weeks, increasing to 0.4mg/kg/day for a further two weeks, with further doubling of the dose at two weekly intervals until seizure-control is obtained, or a maximum of 5mg/kg/day is being given.

In adults on valproate, it is suggested that lamotrigine 25mg be given on alternate days for two weeks, increasing to 25mg daily for two weeks, with further increases at two to four week intervals until seizures are controlled or a maximum dose of 200-400mg is reached. In those who are not receiving valproate, the starting doses can be higher: approximately 2mg/kg/day for children and 25 to 50mg daily in adults. Slow escalation is always important, regardless of co-medication and the starting dose. The plasma level of lamotrigine dose not relate closely to the therapeutic effect; nor, is it useful in the monitoring of adverse events. If the dose is too high, seizure control may deteriorate, after a period of reasonable control. Ataxia and dizziness can occur. Vomiting for no other obvious reason can be an indication that too much lamotrigine is being given.

### Lamotrigine As An Aid To Improved Quality Of Life

As noted above lamotrigine improves control of seizure types which have not responded to previously marketed AEDs. It is also effective, with fewer adverse events for seizures which are responsive to "older" drugs. Lamotrigine dose not cause behavioural difficulties, and many adults have reported a feeling of increased well-being during treatment. However, abolition of frequent sub-clinical seizure discharges, can make the learning disabled person more alert and consequently more active. Thus, improvement in the quality of life of the patient can lead to more difficulties with care and a deterioration in the overall quality of family life. It is important that this is recognised and that provision of appropriate support is available.

## *Vigabatrin*

Vigabatrin is available in tablets, and in sachets containing powder, which can be dissolved in water before administration.

### Treatment Spectrum

The initial trials of vigabatrin were conducted in adults with partial seizures resistant to "older" AEDs. Vigabatrin was shown to be effective (Rimmer & Richens, 1984; Sander & Duncan, 1996). Similarly, in childhood, approximately 50 per cent of those with partial epilepsies can expect at least 50 per cent reduction in seizures, with the introduction of vigabatrin (Dulac, Chiron, Luna, Cusmai, Pajot, Beaumont & Mondragon 1991). Those with symptomatic, rather than cryptogenic, partial seizures did marginally better in the initial studies. However, it is in studies in other seizure types and syndromes, that vigabatrin has shown usefulness of particular interest to those with learning disabilities.

In early studies of the efficacy of vigabatrin in children with many different sorts of seizures, it was noted that those with *infantile spasms* could respond. Therefore, a therapeutic trial of vigabatrin as add-on treatment was initiated (Chiron, Dulac, Beaumont, Palacios, Pajot & Mumford, 1991). Sixty-eight of 70 children who were entered into the trial completed an evaluation period of at least 22 and up to 150 days (mean 96 days), and 46 of the 68 had a greater than 50% reduction in spasms. Clearly, add-on vigabatrin seemed much more effective than any previous therapy. The results were particularly encouraging when the spasms were secondary to tuberous sclerosis; and, those with symptomatic, rather than idiopathic, infantile spasms responded better. A more recent report gives information on vigabatrin when it is given as first-choice monotherapy for infantile spasms (Aicardi, Sabril IS Investigator and Peer Review Groups, Mumford, Dumas & Wood, 1996). The information in this report relates to a retrospective survey of the use, by European doctors, of vigabatrin as the initial treatment. Since this was not a prospective study, the dosage schedules were not standardised. Nevertheless, of the 192 patients who were evaluable, 131 (68 per cent) had an initial response with complete cessation of 'spasms, and a further 37 (19.3 per cent) had a decrease in cluster frequency. Only 23 (12 per cent) of the infants had no change in the frequency of spasms, and only one seemed worse. Seizures of different types, mainly partial, presented after the onset of infantile spasms and during treatment with vigabatrin in 43 (23 per cent) of the 192 children. Twelve of the 43 had recurrences of infantile spasms. An increase in the dose of vigabatrin controlled recurrent infantile spasms in some children, and the later onset partial seizures in some others. At the end of the survey, 96 (50 per cent) of the infants were seizure-free after vigabatrin monotherapy. Once again, infants with tuberous sclerosis were particularly likely to respond. Preliminary data suggests that there are likely to be cognitive advantages in the early control of infantile spasms with vigabatrin, especially in those with tuberous sclerosis (Chiron, Jambaque, Dulac, Pinton, Syrota, 1996).

Treatment of the *Lennox Gastaut syndrome* with vigabatrin has been helpful for some patients, but not others. Of the six patients given vigabatrin by Appleton (1993), none had a significant reduction in any of the presenting seizure types. On the other hand, 85 per cent of 20 children who were given vigabatrin as add-on therapy to valproate experienced a 50 to 100 per cent reduction in seizure frequency (Feucht & Brantner-Intaler,

1994). The seizure types for which the responses were greatest were tonic and atonic; but, atypical absences and tonic-clonic seizures were reduced by 65 per cent and complex partial attacks by 52%. These authors reported an overall increase in myoclonic seizures, but many epileptologists would consider that myoclonic seizures would exclude a diagnosis of Lennox Gastaut Syndrome. The results from another study are also encouraging (Careaga Maldenado, Campos Castello, Fuentes & Dolano, 1995). Fifteen patients with Lennox Gastaut syndrome were given vigabatrin as add-on treatment, usually to valproate, but in some cases to phenobarbitone and/or clobazam. The dose range used was 23-100mg/kg/day. Seven of the 15 patients had more than 50 per cent decreases in seizure frequency, and three of these became seizure-free. No child became worse.

Studies in the rarer epilepsies of early childhood are still awaited, but in a single case of *Landau-Kleffner syndrome*, it has been reported that vigabatrin, when added to carbamazepine, produced a dramatic and almost immediate cessation of seizures and improvement in language abilities (Appleton, Hughes, Beirne & Acomb, 1993). The needs of learning disabled adults were considered at an early stage in the clinical history of vigabatrin (Matilainen, Pitkanen, Ruutiainen, Mervaala, Sarlund & Riekkinen, 1988). Thirty-six patients with *drug-resistant epilepsies* had vigabatrin added to existing therapies for seven months. Almost half, 15 patients, showed a more than 50 per cent decrease in their monthly frequencies of seizures. A further 14 patients had a less effective reduction in seizures, but became more able to join in social activities, were more communicative and their active participation in day-to-day living was better. Of the remaining seven patients, one became psychotic, necessitating withdrawal of vigabatrin early in the study. Studies on the longer-term efficacy of vigabatrin suggest that, overall, up to one-third of patients, may develop tolerance, with resultant poorer seizure control (Sivenius, Ylinen, Murros, Mumford & Reikkinen, 1991). Those with tuberous sclerosis may fare better. If a good response to vigabatrin is obtained in severely learning-disabled patients with tuberous sclerosis, approximately 80 per cent are likely to continue to do well over periods lasting up to three and a half years (Laan, Wefering & Bronwer, 1995).

It is important to characterise the seizures correctly before commencing vigabatrin. Some seizures, including *myoclonia,* as noted in the comments on the Lennox Gastaut syndrome, above, can worsen, or even make a de novo appearance when vigabatrin is introduced (Lortie, Chiron, Mumford & Dulac, 1993). The seizures most likely to become more frequent are generalised and resistant to other therapies; whereas those appearing de novo include partial seizures, which may replace spasms in infants with West syndrome; and myoclonia. Symptomatic infantile spasms have also been reported as a new seizure type after the introduction of vigabatrin. On the other hand, for some patients, complex partial seizures change to simple partial seizures, thus often improving the patient's quality of life. On the whole, changes in the seizure type induced by vigabatrin are considered to be advantageous, rather than producing increased difficulties (Lortie, Chiron, Mumford & Dulac, 1993).

## How To Use Vigabatrin

The dose of vigabatrin can be escalated to maintenance levels within a few days to a week but slower introduction is usual. If the introduction is too rapid, excessive sedation is likely to result. In children the effective maintenance dose is likely to lie between 40 to 100mg/kg/day. Larger doses have been given, particularly for infantile spasms, but there is very little evidence that giving more than 100mg/kg/day leads to any further improvement in seizure control. In infants and children a starting dose of 20 to 30mg/kg/day can be given for three to seven days before doubling the dose to 40 to 60mg/kg/day. If there is no, or an incomplete, response, a further increase in dosage can be made after one to two week. In adults, 500mg, either once or twice daily, is the usual starting dose. Increments in dosage of 500mg per day are made at one to two week intervals to a maximum of between 2G and 3G daily: the maintenance doses for adults usually lie between 1G and 1.5G per day. Vigabatrin is most often given in two divided doses. If renal impairment is present, lower doses should be used. If seizures are going to respond to vigabatrin, they usually do so within the first few weeks of treatment. Thus, prolonged trials at maintenance dosages are not warranted. Vigabatrin should not be stopped abruptly unless this is essential: sudden withdrawal can lead to status epilepticus.

Measurement of vigabatrin plasma levels is not indicated.

## Vigabatrin As An Aid To Improved Quality Of Life

As an effective antiepileptic drug, vigabatrin has an undoubted influence on the quality of life. In addition, for some epilepsies, in particular West syndrome, the cognitive outcome may be better than with other, less effective, medications (Chiron, Jambaque, Dulac, Pinton & Syrota, 1996). There is only one study which reports that vigabatrin may have adverse effects on cognition: slight slowing on a test of motor function and some interference with an aspect of visual memory were recorded (Grunewald, Thompson, Corcoran, Corden, Jackson & Duncan, 1994). Other investigators have not demonstrated any deleterious effect on cognitive abilities (Gilham, Blacklaw, McKee & Brodie, 1993; McGuire, Duncan & Timble, 1992; Mumford, Beaumont & Gisselbrecht,, 1990). In fact, a decrease in the response time on an arithmetical test which relates to central cognitive processing ability was found in one study (McGuire, Duncan & Trimble, 1992).

Behavioural changes can be a major problem with vigabatrin. Up to 10 per cent of patients may develop alterations in mood, such as agitation, irritability, disturbed behaviour or depression (Sander & Duncan, 1996). Up to four per cent become paranoid or psychotic from one to 36 weeks after commencing vigabatrin. Psychosis may occur during a respite from seizures, after a cluster of seizures (Sander & Duncan, 1996), or even after abrupt cessation of treatment with vigabatrin (Brodie & McKee, 1990). Psychosis is very unusual in children, but there is one report of vigabatrin - associated reversible acute psychosis in a seven-year old boy (Martinez, Baines, Marques, Aparisi & Cordon, 1995). Those who have a previous history of depression are most likely to develop depressive symptoms when vigabatrin is introduced (Sander & Duncan, 1996). Clearly, patients who develop psychotic or depressive feelings are not being helped in a general manner, even if their seizures are under better control. Although, reduction of the dosage of vigabatrin may be helpful in some cases, most such patients need to have the dose tapered, with eventual withdrawal.

A further method of assessing whether or not vigabatrin can be helpful is to look at the long-term socio-economic status of treated patients. A ten-year follow-up has been reported (Ylinen, Salmenpera, Clark, Mumford & Reikkinen, 1995). Twenty-two of 56 patients who had an initial good response to vigabatrin were traced after 10 years and their socio-economic circumstances were assessed. Only four were able to work, but epilepsy was not the cause of unemployability in the rest. Two had left institutional care and none had required fresh admission. The overall need for medical care had diminished and six families found that there was a decreased need for supportive involvement by care givers. These findings support the concept that reductions in seizures help other aspects of life.

## Gabapentin

Gabapentin is dispensed in capsules. Currently, it does not have a licence for treatment of children with epilepsy.

## Treatment Spectrum

Almost all of the efficacy studies have been done in patients with resistant partial seizures. Two large multicentre trials have been conducted, using placebo as a comparative agent (UK Gabapentin Study Group, 1990; US Gabapentin Study Group, 1993). In both, 25 or fewer per cent of those receiving gabapentin had reductions in seizure frequency of 50 per cent or more. Eight to ten per cent on placebo had comparable improvements. There was some evidence that patients on higher doses of gabapentin were those most likely to respond. However, in both trials approximately one-fifth of the patients experienced worsening of their seizures. There is anecdotal information which suggests that gabapentin is not helpful for primary generalised seizures and epilepsies. The efficacy of gabapentin in the severe epilepsy syndromes, such as West, Lennox-Gastaut, etc is unknown, but a recent study has reported on experiences in the treatment of developmentally disabled adults (Kerrick, Lott, Anderson & Emery, 1996). Of 32 patients with a mean age of 37 years, 44 per cent had no change in seizure frequency, 28 per cent were worse and 28 per cent had reductions in seizure frequencies of at least 50 per cent. The seizure types present in patients in this study were not identified.

It is clear from the foregoing that gabapentin has made less of an impact on epilepsy than other newer drugs. In a discussion on the place of gabapentin in the therapy of epilepsy, Shorvon (1996) comments that it has little effect on seizure frequency in most patients with severe epilepsy. Thus, it is probable that most of the learning-disabled with epilepsy will need to look to other AEDs for a therapeutic response.

## How To Use Gabapentin

Since gabapentin can be helpful in a minority of patients, the dosage schedule is given. In adults, the dose starts at 400mg daily and is titrated upwards, at weekly intervals, to 1200mg/day, given in three divided doses. Further increments can be given, if considered indicated, to a maximum of 1200mg three times a day (Shorvon, 1996). Withdrawal should be gradual.

## Gabapentin As An Aid To Improved Quality Of Life

For the minority whose seizures are reduced in frequency, gabapentin undoubtedly must improve day-to-day living. Adverse effects are unlikely to interfere with quality of life, since they are largely minor and rarely lead to the need to withdraw gabapentin. No studies of the effects of the use of gabapentin on the activities of day-to-day living have been reported.

## *Topiramate*

Topiramate is dispensed in tablets. There is no liquid formulation. Chewable or dispersible tablets and soluble powders are not available.

### Treatment Spectrum

Topiramate is not licensed in the UK for the treatment of children with epilepsy though a trial in partial seizures in those under 12 years of age is currently in progress.

Information on the use of topiramate in adults with epilepsy is restricted to those who suffer from partial seizures with or without secondary generalisation. Three out of five trials found that more than 40 per cent of patients had more than 50 per cent reductions in their seizure frequencies; in the other two trials 35 and 38 per cent of patients were considered to be responders (Reife, 1996). Thus topiramate could help seizure control in learning-disabled adults whose partial seizures are resistant to other medications. Early cautious, personal experience with topiramate in children suggests that those with resistant partial seizures may also improve, but that they may have unacceptable behavioural side effects.

### How To Use Topiramate

Topiramate should be started at a low dose, with escalation at weekly intervals. The initial dose, 100mg daily, is increased to 100mg twice a day after one week and thereafter by 200mg a week to the effective dose. The maximal recommended dose is 800mg daily. Some patients become unacceptably sleepy at doses which improve seizure control. In these people reduction of the dose may be associated with loss of some of the control: a feature of topiramate which makes it difficult to use in some cases.

### Topiramate As An Aid To Improved Quality Of Life

Reductions in seizure frequency which are achieved with topiramate are undoubtedly an aid to improved life-styles. However, the excessive sleepiness which occurs at higher doses in some patients may detract from control of the seizures. Other central nervous system effects can be even less acceptable. Psychosis has been observed personally and reported from elsewhere: it is not clear which patients are most vulnerable. A young, moderately learning-disabled girl under my care whose seizures were much improved, became withdrawn and ceased to interact with her mother while on topiramate. She was not able to communicate her feelings, secondary to poor linguistic abilities, but became more interactive as topiramate was withdrawn. Clearly, the use of topiramate, which can cause concentration impairment, confusion, and "abnormal thinking" (Reife, 1996) must be very carefully monitored in the learning-disabled.

Topiramate may also be associated with weight loss, which could be a cause for concern in people with poor eating patterns. In addition, renal stones may complicate treatment: a feature which necessitates good fluid intake.

In summary, the place of topiramate in the treatment of epilepsy in those who are not able to verbalise adverse events is still not entirely secure.

## Other Anti-epileptic Drugs

This section includes brief comments on AEDs which do not have licences in the United Kingdom, but which are being used in named patients or in trials.

### Oxcarbazepine

Oxcarbazepine is licensed in Scandinavian countries for the treatment of partial seizures. Its spectrum is very similar to that of carbamazepine, but fewer adverse events and drug interactions are reported. It does, however, have a greater tendency to cause hyponatraemia than carbamazepine, and, for this reason, caution is recommended in its use for elderly patients, and those with cardiac disorders.

### Felbamate

Felbamate was given a great deal of publicity following a trial in the Lennox Gastaut syndrome, conducted in the United States of America (Felbamate Study Group in Lennox-Gastaut Syndrome, 1993). Unfortunately serious systemic side-effects have subsequently restricted its use. In the Lennox-Gastaut syndrome, the total of all astatic seizures in all patients decreased by 44 per cent, with associated decrease in consequent injuries, when felbamate was given. The total numbers of generalised tonic-clonic seizures in all patients fell by 40 per cent, and the total of all seizures by 26 per cent. All these results were significantly better than with placebo. Over 50 per cent of patients had a reduction of more than 50 per cent in astatic seizures, and approximately 50 per cent of all seizures (Dodson, 1993). An open-label study following the initial trial showed that improvements associated with felbamate were sustained for at least 12 months (Dodson, 1993). On the basis of the findings in the Lennox Gastaut syndrome, felbamate was given a licence in the USA. Soon afterwards, reports of aplastic anaemia and hepatic failure associated with treatment with felbamate appeared and in 1994 the general use of felbamate was suspended (Bebin, Sofia & Dreifuss, 1995). In the USA, a licence for selected cases has been retained, but felbamate is not available in Europe.

**Tiagabine**

Tiagabine is being given in trials for both adults and children with partial seizures. A significant reduction in complex partial and secondary generalised seizures, when compared double-blind with placebo, has been reported in adults treated with tiagabine as add-on therapy (Richens, Chadwick, Duncan, Dam, Gram, Mikkelsen, Morrow, Mengel, Shu, McKelvy, Pierce, 1995). Some children who have responded to add-on tiagabine are being continued in a long-term study (Boeliner, Sommerville, Pixton & Lenz, 1996). Withdrawal of other AEDs to achieve tiagabine monotherapy has been achieved in both adults and children (Biton, Alto, Pixton & Sommerville, 1996; Kalviainenen, Salmenpera, Alkia, Mervaaia & Riekkinen, 1996). In clinical trials, tiagabine seems a safe drug, but somnolence and dizziness occur in at least 25 per cent of those treated (Leppik, 1995). The place of tiagabine in the treatment of the learning-disabled with epilepsy is yet to be established.

## Conclusions

New drugs certainly mean there is new hope for the control of epilepsy in the learning-disabled. In particular, the treatment of infantile-spasms with vigabatrin and of the Lennox-Gastaut syndrome with lamotrigine have reduced morbidity in both these conditions. Reductions in the frequencies of seizures associated with sudden loss of posture make injuries less likely, and have implications for the amount of supervision required. Thus the amount of independence allowed and the subsequent freedom from constant care can improve the lives of care-givers as well as those of learning-disabled people. When introducing new drugs, it is important to be aware that learning-disabled people may have difficulty in communicating unpleasant effects, especially those which cause alterations in thought processes. Particular vigilance is necessary.

## References

Aicardi, J., Sabril, I. S., Investigator and Peer Review Groups, Mumford, J. P., Dumas, C. & Wood, S. (1996). Vigabatrin as initial therapy for infantile spasms: A European retrospective survey. *Epilepsia,* 37, 638-642.

Appleton, R.E. (1993). The role of vigabatrin in the management of infantile epileptic syndromes. *Neurology,* 43 (suppl5) S21-S23.

Appleton, R., Hughes, A., Beirne, M. & Acomb, B. (1993). Vigabatrin in the Landau-Kleffner Syndrome. *Developmental Medicine and Child Neurology,* 35, 457-458.

Bebin, E.M., Sofia, R.D., Dreifuss, F.E. (1995). Felbamate: toxicity. In: Levy, R.H., Mattson, R.H. & Meldrum, B.S. (edss) *Antiepileptic Drugs, Fourth Edition,* New York, Raven Press, pp. 823-827.

Besag, F. (1992). Lamotrigine: paediatric experience. In: Richens, A. (ed.), *International Clinical Practice Series, Clinical Update on Lamotrigine: A Novel Antiepileptic Agent.* Wells Medical Limited, Royal Tunbridge Wells, pp 53-60.

Besag, F.M.C., Wallace, S.J., Dulac, O., Alving, J., Spencer, S.C., & Hosking, G. (1995). Lamotrigine for the treatment of epilepsy in childhood. *Journal of Pediatrics,* 127, 991-997.

Billard, C., Motte, J., Arvidsson, D., Trevathan, E., Talladai, M., Campos, J. & Douglas, C. (1996). Double-blind, placebo-controlled evaluation of the safety and efficacy of lamotrigine (Lamictal) for the treatment of patients with a clinical diagnosis of Lennox-Gastaut Syndrome. *Epilepsia,* 37 (suppl 4), 92.

Biton, V., Alto, G.H., Pixton, G.C. & Sommerville, K.W. (1996). Tiagabine monotherapy in adults and children in a long-term study. *Epilepsia,* 37 (suppl 5), 167

Boeliner, S.W., Sommerville, K.W., Pixton, G.C. & Lenz, G.T. (1996). Long-term treatment of children with tiagabine. *Epilepsia,* 37 (suppl 5), 168.

Brodie, M.J. (1992). Lamotrigine. *Lancet,* 339, 1397-1400

Brodie, M.J. & McKee, P.J.W. (1990). Vigabatrin and psychosis. *Lancet,* 335, 1279.

Brodie, M.J., Richens, A & Yuen, A.W.C. (1995). Double-blind comparison of lamotrigine and carbamazepine in newly diagnosed epilepsy. *Lancet,* 345, 476-479.

Careaga Maldonada, J., Campos Castello, J., Fuentes, E.G.U. & Bolario, R.P. (1995). Vigabatrin in the management of Lennox-Gastaut Syndrome. *Epilepsia,* 36 (suppl 3), S102.

Chiron, C., Dulac, O., Beaumont, D., Palacios, L., Pajot, N. & Mumford, J. (1991). Therapeutic trial of vigabatrin in refractory infantile spasms. *Journal of Child Neurology*, 6 (suppl 2), 2S52-2S59.

Chiron, C., Jambaque, I., Dulac, O., Pinton, F. & Syrota, A. (1996). Functional imaging SPECT and neuropsychological evaluation of paediatric patients during the course of West Syndrome. *Epilepsie-Blatter*, 9, 8.

Dodson, W.E., (1993). Felbamate in the treatment of Lennox-Gastaut Syndrome: Results of a 12-month open-label study following a randomized clinical trial. *Epilepsia*, 34 (suppl 7), S18-S24.

Dulac, O., Chiron, C., Luna, D., Cusmai, R., Pajot, N., Beaumont, D., & Modragon, S. (1991). Vigabatrin in childhood epilepsy. *Journal of Child Neurology*, 6 (suppl), 2S30-2S37.

Felbamate Study Group in Lennox-Gastaut Syndrome (1993). Efficacy of felbamate in childhood epileptic encephalopathy (Lennox-Gastaut Syndrome). *New England Journal of Medicine*, 328, 29-33.

Feucht, M. & Brantner-Inthaler, S. (1994). Gamma-Vinyl-GABA (vigabatrin) in the therapy of Lennox-Gastaut Syndrome: An open study. *Epilepsia*, 35, 993-998.

Gillham, R.A., Blacklaw, J., McKee, P.J.W., & Brodie, M.J. (1993). Effect of vigabatrin on sedation and cognitive function in patients with refractory epilepsy. *Journal of Neurology, Neurosurgery and Psychiatry*, 56, 1271-1275.

Grunewald, R.A., Thompson, P.J., Corcoran, P.S., Corden, Z., Jackson, G.D. & Duncan J.S. (1994). Effects of vigabatrin on partial seizures and cognitive function. *Journal of Neurology, Neurosurgery and Psychiatry*, 57, 1057-1063.

Gusev, E., Petroukhin, A., Bourd, G., Medvedev, M. & Mukhin, K. (1996). Lamotrigine (Lamictal) in treatment of resistant epilepsy in children. *Epilepsia*, 37 (suppl 4), 67.

Kalviainen, R., Salmenpera,T., Aikia, M., Mervaala, E., & Reikkinen, P.J. (1996). Tiagabine monotherapy in chronic partial epilepsy. *Epilepsia*, 37 (suppl 5), 167.

Kerrick, J.M., Lott, R.S., Anderson, K. & Emery, M. (1996). Experience with gabapentin in developmentally disabled adults with refractory seizures: adverse effects and efficacy outcomes. *Epilepsia*, 37 (suppl 5), 161.

Laan, L.A.E.M., v.d. Wetering, B.L. & Brouwer, O.F. (1995). Long-term effects of vigabatrin in patients with tuberous sclerosis. *Epilepsia*, 36 (suppl 3), S107.

Leppik, I.E. (1995). Tiagabine: The safety landscape. *Epilepsia*, 36 (suppl 6), 36 (suppl 6), S10-S13.

Lortie, A., Chiron, C., Mumford, J. & Dulac, O. (1993). The potential for increasing seizure frequency, relapse and appearance of new seizure types with vigabatrin. *Neurology*, 43 (suppl 5), S24-S27.

McGuire, A.M., Duncan, J.S. & Trimble, M.R. (1992). Effects of vigabatrin on cognitive function and mood, when used as add-on therapy in patients with intractable epilepsy. *Epilepsia*, 33, 128-134.

Manonmani V. & Wallace, S.J. (1994). Epilepsy with myoclonic absences. *Archives of Disease in Childhood*, 70, 288-290.

Martinez, A.C., Baines, J.P.O., Marques, M.B., Aparisi, A.E. & Cordon, F.G. (1995). Vigabatrin - associated reversible acute psychosis in a child. *Annals of Pharmacotherapy*, 29, 115-117.

Matilainen, R., Pitkanen, A., Runtiainen, T., Mervaala, E., Sarhind, H. & Reikkinen, P. (1988). Effect of vigabatrin on epilepsy in mentally retarded parients: A 7- month follow-up study. *Neurology*, 38, 743-747.

Mumford, J.P., Beaumont, D. & Gisselbrecht, D. (1990). Cognitive function, mood and behaviour in vigabatrin treated parients. *Acta Neurologica Scandinavica,* 82 (suppl 133), 15.

Oller, L.F.V., Russi, A., & Oller Daurella, L. (1991). Lamotrigine in the Lennox-Gastaut syndrome. *Epilepsia,* 32 (suppl 1), 58.

Reife, R.A. (1996). Topiramate. In: Shorvon, S.D., Dreifuss, F.E., Fish, D. & Thomas, D. (Eds). *The Treatment of Epilepsy*, Oxford, Blackwell Science, pp. 471-481.

Richens, A., Chadwick, D.W., Duncan, J.S., Dam, M., Gram, L. Mikkelsen, M., Morrow, J., Mengel, H., Shu, V., McKelvy, J.F. & Pierce, M.W. (1995). Adjunctive treatment of partial seizures with tiagabine: A placebo-controlled trial. *Epilepsy Research*, 21, 37-42.

Rimmer, E.M. & Richens, A. (1984). Double-blind study of gamma-vinyl GABA in patients with refractory epilepsy. *Lancet*, ii, 189-190.

Sander, J.W.A.S & Duncan, J.S. (1996). Vigabatrin. In: Shorvon, S.D., Dreifuss, F.E., Fish, D. & Thomas, D. (Eds*). The Treatment of Epilepsy,* Oxford, Blackwell Science, pp 491-499.

Santavouri, P., Himberg, J.J., Ahola, A., Hosking, G. & Yuen, A.W.C. (1995). Lamotrigine Therapy in infantile neuronal ceriod lipofuscinosis. *Epilepsia*, 36 (suppl 3), S264.

Schlumberger, E., Chavez, F., Palacios, L., Rey E., Pajot, N. & Dulac, O. (1994). Lamotrigine in treatment of 120 children with epilepsy. *Epilepsia*,     35, 359-367.

Shorvon, S.D. (1996). Gabapentin. In: Shorvon, S.D., Dreifuss, F.E., Fish, D. & Thomas, D. (Eds). *The Treatment of Epilepsy*, Oxford, Blackwell Science, pp 429-437.

Sivenius, J., Ylinen, A., Murros, K., Mumford, J.P. & Reikkinen, P.J. (1991). Vigabatrin in drug resistant partial epilepsy: a 5 year follow-up study. *Neurology*, 41, 562-556.

Timmings, P.L. & Richens, A. (1992). Lamotrigine as an add-on drug in the management of Lennox-Gastaut Syndrome. *European Neurology,* 32, 305-307.

UK Gabapentin Study Group (1990). Gabapentin in partial epilepsy. *Lancet*, i, 1114-1117.

US Gabapentin Study Group (1993). Gabapentin therapy in refractory epilepsy: A double-blind placebo-controlled parallel group study. *Neurology*, 43, 2292-2298.

Wallace, S.J. (1989). Lamotrigine in resistant childhood epilepsy. *Neuropediatrics*, 20, 16.

Wallace, S.J. (1993). Lamotrigine: useful therapy for astatic seizures. *Neuropediatrics*, 24, 72.

Wallace, S.J. (1994). Lamotrigine - a clinical overview. *Seizure,* 3 (suppl A), 47-51.

Ylinen, A., Salmenpera, T., Clark, T., Mumford, J. & Reikkinen, P.J. (1995). Effect of 10 years of vigabatrin therapy on socioeconomic status. *Epilepsia*, 36 (suppl 5), S107.

**Sheila Wallace** is a consultant paediatric neurologist at the University Hospital of Wales.

**Contact Address**
University Hospital of Wales
Cardiff, CF4 4XW
Wales

# 11
## *Genetics and Learning Disability*

## Anita Thapar and Peter McGuffin

It has long been known that there are many different causes of learning disabilities. Often learning disability has been sub-divided into two groups on the basis of IQ test scores. It has commonly been considered that for individuals with *mild* learning disability, psycho-social factors such as social disadvantage were primary contributory factors whereas *moderate to severe* learning disability was thought to be explained mainly by genetic disorders and identifiable biological insults such as infections and birth trauma.

However, it is becoming increasingly apparent that these two groups are not completely distinct. We now know that mild learning disability can have a biological basis and that a definite cause is not always identified for severe learning disability.

In recent years there have been tremendous advances in genetics research which have been accompanied by increasing scientific and public interest in the subject. Progress in genetics research is of course particularly important in the field of learning disabilities as many genetic syndromes are associated with learning disability. New research techniques are enabling scientists to locate genes for an increasing number of genetic syndromes. Although these represent important advances, it is important to remember that genetic syndromes resulting from specific genes or chromosome defects are not only rare in the general population but that most learning disability is not attributable to such syndromes.

Genetics research is now also being used to understand more about the genetic basis of more common disorders such as diabetes, schizophrenia as well as normal behaviour and traits such as personality and intelligence. We call these disorders and traits *complex* because they can not be explained by a defect in one particular gene and because environmental factors are also important.

In this chapter we will start by giving an overview of the most important types of genetic conditions associated with learning disability. We will then explain current research methods being used to understand the genetic basis of complex disorders and traits and discuss the possible impact that the findings from this research might have on the field of learning disabilities.

## Overview of Genetics

The human body is made up of millions of cells each of which contains a genetic blueprint which we pass onto our children. The genetic information in our cells is carried on **chromosomes**, of which humans have 23 pairs.

Chromosomes have a long arm and a short arm and stain in bands when dyed. One set of 23 is inherited from the father and the other from the mother. One of the 23 chromosome pairs consists of sex chromosomes which determine the sex of a child. Females have two X chromosomes, whereas males have one X chromosome and one Y chromosome. The remaining 22 chromosome pairs are called autosomes.

Our genetic information is coded in **genes**. Humans have about one hundred thousand genes which lie along the length of the chromosomes. The position of the gene on a chromosome is called a locus. Genes code for characteristics such as eye colour by means of their special structure. Genes consist of a substance called deoxyribo-nucleic-acid, **DNA**, which is made up of **nucleotide bases**. There are four types of nucleotide bases (cytosine, guanine, adenine and thymine) which are very important as the coding message in genes lies in the sequence of these bases (see Figure 1).

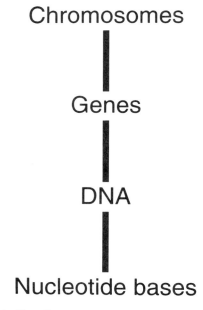

# Chromosomes

# Genes

# DNA

# Nucleotide bases

*Figure 1: How Human Genetic Information is Carried*

We will now describe some of the most common genetic defects associated with learning disability.

## Single Gene Disorders

Single gene disorders are characterised by a defect within a particular gene and are rare. However they are important in that they tend to be serious conditions, clinically distinctive and are often associated with learning disability. There are approximately 210 single gene disorders which are known to be associated with learning disability. These single gene disorders can be sub-divided into two main groups, namely, autosomal disorders and sex-linked disorders.

### Autosomal Disorders

Autosomal disorders are so called because the defective gene lies on an autosome. These disorders can be inherited in either a **dominant** or **recessive** fashion. For autosomal dominant conditions (e.g. tuberous sclerosis) only one defective gene needs to be inherited from a parent for the child to show the disorder, whereas for autosomal recessive conditions (e.g. phenylketonuria), a faulty gene needs to be inherited from both mother and father. These disorders often show a characteristic pattern of clinical features, affecting appearance, pattern of learning disability and associated features such as epilepsy or physical disorder. Many cases have a well recognised pattern of biochemical abnormalities. Also for many of these conditions the responsible genes have been localised, that is we know where and on which chromosome the gene lies. Advances in research techniques, which we will describe later, have resulted in the localisation of an increasing number of genes responsible for single gene disorders.

### X-linked Disorders

In X-linked conditions the genetic defect is localised on the X chromosome. These disorders are usually commoner in boys because, as mentioned earlier, males have one X chromosome and one Y chromosome whereas females have two X chromosomes. Thus, for an X-linked recessive condition, a female would need to inherit two abnormal X chromosomes to show the disorder, whereas males only need one abnormal X chromosome to show the condition. This is because the Y chromosome does not compensate for the defective gene on the X.

It was recognised very early that learning disability is commoner among males than females. This indirectly suggested that X-linked disorders might be an important cause of learning disability. Indeed we now know of a large number of X-linked conditions which are associated with learning disability and many of these have been mapped onto specific locations on the X chromosome. It has been estimated that there are approximately 105 X-linked disorders where learning disability is a primary characteristic, and of these 53 genes have been mapped onto a location on the X chromosome. The commonest and best known X-linked disorder associated with learning disability is Fragile X syndrome which shows a particularly interesting pattern of inheritance.

**Fragile X Syndrome** Fragile X is the single most common known inherited cause of learning disability. It affects approximately 1 in 2000 to 1 in 3000 people. Fragile X syndrome was named as such because the condition is characterised by the presence of a so called fragile site on the X chromosome. This fragile site is a band located on the long arm of chromosome X (the location site is labeled Xq27.3) which does not stain with dye.

Previously the diagnosis of Fragile X syndrome was based on the finding of this fragile site. However, presence of this fragile site is not always a reliable marker of Fragile X syndrome. In recent years, as the gene for fragile X has been found, it is now possible to accurately confirm a diagnosis of Fragile X syndrome by using molecular testing. The characteristic features of this condition include learning disability, macro orchidism (large testes), large ears and a long face (see also the chapter by O'Brien in this volume).

Until recently the inheritance pattern of Fragile X syndrome was thought to be extremely puzzling. Firstly, it was observed that apparently normal fathers seemed to be able to transmit the syndrome to apparently normal daughters who then produced affected male children. The second unusual observation was that the severity of the syndrome appears to increase from one generation to the next. However because of recent molecular genetic research findings, we now understand the biological basis to these observations.

The gene responsible for the Fragile X syndrome which has now been identified is known as FMR-1. As mentioned earlier, genes code for characteristics by means of a coding sequence of nucleotide bases. It has now been found that within the Fragile X gene there is a repeat sequence of three nucleotides (trinucleotide repeat = cytosine, guanine, guanine -CGG). All of us have between 6 and 54 copies of this CGG repeat. However, Fragile X carriers (carriers are individuals who are carrying a faulty gene and can pass it onto their children but who do not show the disorder) show a longer sequence of repeats. Once this repeat sequence gets longer it becomes unstable and shows a tendency to increase further in size when transmitted to the next generation. However, this increase in size from one generation to the next only seems to happen when the gene is transmitted by a female and not a male. It seems that when the repeat sequence reaches a critical length (about 200 copies) individuals will then show the features of Fragile X syndrome.

The discovery of this type of abnormally long repeat sequence, otherwise known as "heritable, unstable DNA" explains why the disorder becomes progressively more severe with subsequent generations (this is known as anticipation) and why it seems to make a difference as to whether the defect is transmitted by a male or by a female. We now know that unstable repeat sequences within other genes are responsible for many other genetic conditions, such as Huntingdon's Chorea and Myotonic Dystrophy disorders which also show anticipation.

## Chromosomal Abnormalities

Chromosomal abnormalities can be divided into two main types. Firstly, those where there is a change in the **number** of chromosomes, and secondly, those where there is a change in the **structure** of chromosomes, for example, deletion (one bit of a chromosome is missing), and translocations (a bit of one chromosome has broken off and become attached to or changes place with another chromosome).

Recently, more sophisticated laboratory techniques are allowing us to detect very small deletions, known as submicroscopic deletions, which would not previously have been detected. Chromosomal abnormalities explain up to 40% of severe and between 10-20% of mild learning disability. Although chromosomal abnormalities are **genetic** abnormalities, it is important to remember that these abnormalities are not necessarily **inherited**, that is these defects are not necessarily passed on from one generation to the next. In fact, we know that most chromosomal abnormalities arise spontaneously and those leading to an alteration in number of chromosomes e.g. Down Syndrome occur more commonly to older mothers.

### Down Syndrome

Down syndrome is the commonest form of learning disability caused by chromosomal abnormality and occurs in approximately 1 in 1000 births.

Down syndrome is caused by an extra copy of chromosome 21 which nearly always arises spontaneously and thus although genetic, it is not usually inherited. This is except for a minority (approximately 2%) where Down syndrome is caused by a chromosomal translocation which may be carried by one or other of the parents. Although the clinical features of Down syndrome are well known and highly characteristic, we still do not understand exactly how these clinical features arise and which particular genes on chromosome 21 contribute.

One area of interest has been suggested by findings of post mortem studies which show that nearly all those with Down syndrome by their mid-40's show brain changes characteristic of Alzheimer's disease. We know that some cases of early onset Alzheimer's disease are caused by defects in a gene on chromosome 21 which provides the recipe for a protein known as amyloid precursor protein (APP). It has been suggested that the reason for the Alzheimer-like brain changes in Down syndrome is because those with Down syndrome will have an extra copy of the APP gene. However, other research suggests that a different region of the chromosome (band q22) is critical for the typical features of Down syndrome, namely, learning disability, heart defects and facial changes and the APP gene is not within this region. It is hoped that as more genes are found on chromosome 21 we will understand more about the biological basis of Down syndrome.

## Other Genetic Conditions

We will mention two other genetic conditions, Prader-Willi syndrome and Angelman syndrome, because of their interesting pattern of inheritance. Both of these syndromes are examples of disorders that may arise because of a recently discovered type of subtle chromosomal anomaly resulting from a tiny deletion (microdeletion) of part of a chromosome. Furthermore they show another rather surprising, newly discovered phenomenon called **imprinting**.

### Prader-Willi Syndrome

Individuals affected by Prader-Willi syndrome characteristically show obesity, short stature, small hands and feet, almond shaped eyes, squint, and a tendency to eat excessively. Approximately 40% show learning disability. The condition is rare and it only occurs in approximately 1 in 25,000 people. Although it is a genetic condition, most cases are sporadic rather than familial.

The genetics of Prader-Willi syndrome is particularly interesting in that it illustrates the fact that for some disorders, it makes a difference as to which parent the defect is inherited from. The critical defect is a deletion on the short arm of chromosome 15 (15q11-13). However, it seems that the features of Prader-Willi syndrome are only exhibited when this deletion occurs on the chromosome 15 which is inherited from the **father**. It now appears that approximately 70% of reported cases of Prader-Willi syndrome show this deletion which originates from the father.

A similar type of deletion arising on a chromosome 15 which is inherited from the mother appears to be associated with Angelman syndrome. The features of this condition are entirely different, as described below.

This phenomenon of different expression of genes according to whether they come from the mother or the father is now termed **genomic imprinting**. The evidence of this being important for Prader-Willi syndrome is further supported by the observation that in rare circumstances where chromosomes become jumbled in such a way that both chromosomes 15 are inherited from the mother (instead of one from the mother and one from the father) this also results in cases of Prader-Willi syndrome.

### Angelman Syndrome

Angelman syndrome is again rare, in that it only affects approximately 1 in 20,000 individuals and most cases are sporadic. Affected individuals show severe learning disability, jerky movements, fits and unprovoked laughter. As mentioned earlier, the critical defect is a deletion on the chromosome 15 (15q11-13) which is inherited from the **mother**. Angelman syndrome can also arise when both chromosomes 15 are inherited from the father (3% of cases). Thus, for Angelman syndrome it seems the critical problem is the absence of this region on maternally derived chromosome 15.

Although we now know which region of the chromosome is involved and have laboratory methods of testing for these conditions, the gene or genes within the critical region of the chromosome have yet to be actually identified.

## Multi-factorial Disorders and Traits

Although when considering the genetics of learning disability the temptation is to focus on single gene defects and chromosomal abnormalities, it is important to remember that most learning disability is not accounted for by these disorders. For a very large proportion of those with learning disability there is no recognisable specific cause. Although some of these individuals may later be found to have a previously undetected chromosomal abnormality or single gene defect, there will remain a substantial proportion for whom there is no recognisable specific cause. It is generally assumed that for this group, the learning disability is likely to have been influenced by a number of different **susceptibility genes** as well as by **environmental factors**.

This type of inheritance is known as multi-factorial transmission and probably best describes the inheritance of most common types of complex disorder, such as heart disease, diabetes, schizophrenia and asthma. There is also evidence that normal traits such as weight, height, blood pressure and IQ are best viewed as multi-factorial traits.

It has been suggested that learning disability, when there is no identifiable cause, should be considered as representing the lower end of the normal IQ distribution. That is we should consider that the factors which influence this group of learning disability are the same as those that influence intelligence. There has been much interest in the genetics of intelligence and although some research has been controversial, there are now some very consistent findings.

In general it appears that biologically related relatives, for example brothers and sisters, parents and children, show much more similarity for IQ than unrelated individuals. Further work, for example twin studies and adoption studies (see McGuffin et al, 1994 for explanations) show three main findings.

Firstly, it has been consistently found that genetic factors influence intelligence.

However, the second main group of findings suggest that environmental effects are also important, particularly in childhood. For example, it seems that the mean IQ of children born in socially disadvantaged families but raised in middle class homes is considerably higher than the IQ of their biological brothers and sisters who continue to be raised in the socially disadvantaged homes. In general, it appears that the environmental factors of most importance in influencing IQ are those environmental factors which are not shared by members of the same family. An example of this type of environmental factor would be a head injury experienced by one member of a family.

The third group of findings suggests that the influence of genetic factors seems to increase in importance as people get older, whereas the effect of family factors seems to be most important in childhood. Overall, although we know that both genetic and environmental factors influence intelligence, as yet it remains unknown as to which particular genes are influential and by and large which environmental factors are the most important.

## Molecular Genetics Research

The main success of modern molecular genetics has been in identifying and localising genes responsible for conditions that we know are genetically influenced. There have been major successes in identifying an increasing number of genes responsible for single gene conditions such as phenylketoneuria. However, these single gene conditions show predictable patterns of inheritance (i.e., autosomal dominant, recessive or X-linked).

Although these are important advances, these conditions are of course rare within the general population. The real challenge remains in identifying genes which cause much more common conditions, such as heart disease. Understanding the genetic basis of these sorts of conditions is much more difficult, in that they do not show characteristic patterns of inheritance and as mentioned earlier are generally considered as multi-factorial conditions. However, we now have the techniques for identifying susceptibility genes for these so called complex disorders.

### Markers and Genetic Maps

The main basis of these advances is that we now have the technology for developing a very large number of informative genetic markers. These genetic markers can be thought of as sign posts along chromosomes. Just as it is easier to locate a small village using a detailed map which has many reference points marked on it, it is easier to find a gene when we have a genetic map with many markers at close intervals along the chromosome. As more and more markers are being mapped onto the human gene, we have an increasingly informative and useful "genetic map".

The existence of this genetic map, the relative ease with which we can now manufacture markers and other laboratory techniques which speed up previously laborious processes are now enabling us to successfully locate an increasing number of disease genes.

The essential principle of locating a disease gene is illustrated in Figure 2. In this figure, we have represented a stretch of chromosome along which we have five markers, A, B, C, D, and E. The research methods described below essentially allow us to find out where the disease gene X is by the process of finding out that the disease gene is very near to marker C. In this very simple hypothetical example we have shown five markers. Markers exist in different forms and these vary from person to person. So, for example, marker A could exist in three various forms, e.g. A1, A2 or A3. These variants are termed alleles.

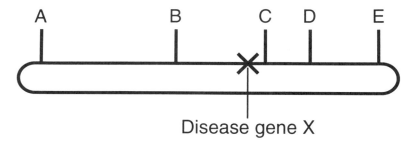

*Figure 2: Locating a Diseased Gene*

### Finding a gene

There are a number of research methods which are currently used to detect and localise genes.

**Linkage studies**    As mentioned earlier, for every pair of chromosomes a child inherits one chromosome from the father and one from the mother. Before these chromosomes are then passed on to his own child, the chromosome from the father and the chromosome from the mother will cross over, as shown in Figure 3. This process is called **recombination** which essentially means that genes along the chromosome get shuffled around and the relative location of one gene to another changes.

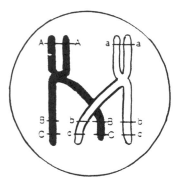

*Figure 3: Crossing over or Recombination*

Of course, for two genes that are close together on a chromosome these will tend to get transmitted together. If they are extremely close together they will be transmitted together for many generations as it is unlikely that they will be split apart by recombination. If a disease and a marker gene are co-transmitted in families significantly more than you would expect by chance, this is known as **linkage**. This is another way of saying that, that particular marker gene seems to be close to the location of the disease gene.

Thus, in linkage studies the basic approach consists of collecting families where many different members are affected by the disease that one is interested in. We then examine many markers and test whether the disease is linked with any of the markers. As we now have many markers available it is now possible to do a whole genome search (a search along every single chromosome at regular intervals) when looking for linkage.

If we find evidence for linkage, we need to apply a statistical test to check whether the finding might have arisen by chance. The real test of whether we have found the disease gene is if the same results can be found in another study; that is we need replication.

Although linkage methods have been very successful in finding genes for single gene disorders, there are a number of problems with using them in studies of complex multi-factorial disorders such as diabetes and schizophrenia. One of the main problems is that for these complex disorders we do not know the mode of inheritance (e.g., autosomal recessive or dominant). Therefore a method which is commonly used in linkage studies of complex disorders is the affected sib pair method.

**Affected sib pair linkage studies**   In affected sib pair studies, rather than collecting whole families the approach is to collect siblings (brothers and sisters) where both siblings have the disease that we are studying. Brothers and sisters inherit their genes from the same parents (although not necessarily the same genes unless they are identical twins) and therefore if we look at the patterns of their markers we would expect them to share some but not all of the marker alleles in common. If the marker allele is linked to the disease we would expect that brothers and sisters who both have the disease will also share that type of marker allele more often than would be expected. This type of affected sib pair strategy enabled researchers to find susceptibility genes for diseases such as insulin dependent diabetes and this approach is now being used in large studies searching for genes for disorders such as schizophrenia and autism.

So far we have focused on linkage methods for finding genes where we collect multiply affected family members. Although linkage studies are very useful, the only problem is that they are not very good at detecting genes where the effect is very small. For many complex disorders it could be that there are multiple susceptibility genes each of only small effect and thus it is possible they will not be detected using linkage approaches. Also it is not always easy to collect families where multiple members have the same disorder. Another type of approach which is more sensitive in locating genes of small effect is called an association study.

**Association studies**    An association approach involves collecting a sample of people all of whom have a particular disease and a control group, that is a sample of people who are well and who do not have the disease. Different markers are then compared between the group with the disease and the group who are well. If one particular marker allele is significantly more common in the ill group compared to the well group this suggests that that marker allele is **associated** with the disease.

Once positive association has been found we need to consider the possible reasons for this association. There are three main explanations for association.

Firstly, it may be that the associated marker allele is actually contributing to the cause of the disease.

Secondly, it may be that the marker allele is extremely close to the disease susceptibility gene. This situation is known as **linkage disequilibrium**.

The third reason is that the control group might differ from the group with the disease in some other way, that is inadvertently we might have chosen two groups who were not really comparable at least at a genetic level. This artifact which is not a true association is known as population stratification and can unfortunately cause problems. For example, a number of studies of different psychiatric disorders found what appeared to be association but these findings were not replicated and appeared to be due to population stratification.

However, previous criticisms of association studies are now being overcome by using a technique whereby genetic information from the parents is used as a control. Although association studies are very powerful and can detect small genetic effects, there are drawbacks to this method. One of the main difficulties is that association will only be detected if the marker allele is extremely close to the disease gene. Unlike linkage studies, if the marker allele is some distance away from the disease gene, association will not be detected.

For this reason, in general, for association studies rather than using lots of markers and doing a total genome screen we only use selected markers in genes which we think are likely to be involved in the disease process. These are known as "candidate genes". However for disorders such as psychiatric disorders where we do not fully understand the disease process, it can be difficult to choose suitable candidate genes.

**Quantitative trait loci**   So far we have focused on looking for genes for medical disorders.  However there is also  very good evidence that lots of normal traits such as personality, weight, height and IQ are genetically influenced.   Unlike medical conditions which we consider people either have or don't have these sorts of normal traits are **quantities** of which people have a certain amount, such as  kilogrammes of weight. Another less obvious example is if we ask people to complete personality questionnaires we could obtain scores of how 'extroverted' they are. These sorts of traits are often known as **quantitative traits**.

A decade ago there was considerable interest when genes for quantitative traits in the tomato plant were identified.  A number of different genes were identified and localised which were found to influence certain quantitative characteristics of a tomato, such as pH and size.

This approach is now being used to find genes which influence human quantitative traits such as personality, intelligence and blood pressure. These types of studies are known as quantitative trait loci or QTL studies.

In general it is again assumed that there will be a number of genes as well as environmental factors which influence these traits. Although as yet there have been few results reported from human QTL  studies there are some interesting findings emerging.  For example, there was recent interest when a dopamine D4 receptor gene polymorphism (a gene coding for a receptor in the brain which is thought to be important in human behaviour) was found to be associated with personality measures of sensation seeking. Sensation seeking people tend to be more adventurous and enjoy excitement and novelty.  This result was found in two separate studies, one in Israel and one in the United States.  It remains to be seen whether this finding can be further replicated and whether other such findings for different quantitative measures emerge.

## *Conclusions and Implications*

The advances in genetics research  have been rapid and are having a major impact on the field of learning disability. Identification of chromosomal abnormalities and genes responsible for single gene conditions are important in terms of understanding more about what causes a person's disability, for prenatal testing and genetic counselling. The real challenge in the future lies in understanding more about the causes of other, commoner forms of learning disability, detecting genes of smaller effect and in unraveling the effects of genes and environment.

## Further Reading

McGuffin, P., Owen, M.J., O'Donovan, M.C., Thapar, A. & Gottesman, I.I. (1994). *Seminars in Psychiatric Genetics*. London: Gaskell.

Plomin, R., DeFries, J.C. & McClearn, G.E. (1990*). Behavioral Genetics: A Primer*. New York: Freeman.

Simonoff,E., Bolton, P. & Rutter, M. (1996). Mental retardation: genetic findings, clinical implications and research agenda. *Journal of Child Psychology and Psychiatry*, 37, 259-280.

Thapar, A., Gottesman, I.I., Owen, M.J., O'Donovan, M.C., & McGuffin, P. (1994). The genetics of mental retardation. *British Journal of Psychiatry*, 164, 747-758.

### Acknowledgements

We would like to thank Dr. Jill Clayton-Smith, Department of Clinical Genetics, St. Mary's Hospital, Manchester for her comments.

**Anita Thapar** is Senior Lecturer and Consultant Child Psychiatrist at the University of Manchester. She trained in genetics research whilst a Medical Research Council (MRC) Fellow in Cardiff. Her current research is on psychiatric and developmental genetics in childhood.

**Peter McGuffin** is Professor and Head of the Division of Psychological Medicine at University of Wales, College of Medicine. He was previously an MRC Senior Fellow at the Institute of Psychiatry, London. His long-standing research interest is in the genetics of normal and abnormal behaviour.

### Contact Addresses

Department of Child & Adolescent Psychiatry,
Royal Manchester Children's Hospital, Pendlebury,
Manchester. M27 4HA, England

Department of Psychological Medicine,
University of Wales College of Medicine,
Heath Park, Cardiff. CF4 4XN, Wales

# 12
# *Behavioural Phenotypes*

## Gregory O'Brien

In this chapter I aim to provide a general introduction to behavioural phenotypes. The chapter begins with a description and explanation of the behavioural phenotype and its importance. This is discussed with reference to a few key conditions of interest in behavioural phenotypy. There follows a brief account of clinical approaches to measurement of behavioural phenotypes. Some of the recent research findings in the field are then summarised with respect to certain syndromes commonly encountered in clinical work with people with learning disabilities/mental retardation.

### *The Behavioural Phenotype Concept*

In many ways, it is easier to say what we do not mean by "behavioural phenotype" than what we do mean. For in saying that a given syndrome or cause of learning disability has a behavioural phenotype we are not proposing that all individuals affected by the condition in question will have all of the behaviours in question. This is crucially important. The essence of the behavioural phenotype concept was captured at the first meeting of the society for the study of behavioural phenotypes (SSBP, 1990*):*

*"that some of the behaviours exhibited by children with biologically based mentally handicapping disorders are organically determined".*

Here, it is emphasised that many other influences - developmental, biological and environmental- operate in complex interactions between and constantly shape those behaviours which are a biological result of the genetic syndrome in question.

A useful definition of behavioural phenotype was proposed by Flint and Yule (1993).

*"The behavioural phenotype is a characteristic pattern of motor, cognitive, linguistic and social abnormalities which is consistently associated with a biological disorder. In some cases, the behavioural phenotype may constitute a psychiatric disorder; in others, behaviours which are not usually regarded as symptoms of psychiatric diagnoses may occur."*

The behavioural phenotype comprises the common, characteristic behavioural findings of a given syndrome. In this definition no simple pathway is envisaged as link between behavioural phenotype and the associated gene(s), or genotype. On the contrary, if our understanding of the increasingly complex manner in which genetic influences result in phenotypes is on target, the links are more like spaghetti than simple straight pathways: tangled up, often difficult to see, but there for the extraction given due care and attention.

It is useful to recognise two ways to approach genotype-phenotype links: one starting at the gene end (genomic) and one at the phenotype/behaviour end (phenomic).

**Genomic**    In the genomic approach one studies genetically identifiable conditions, and seeks to identify to what extent there are behavioural characteristics of the condition.    It was work of this type which first led Nyhan to ascribe a severely mutilating and refractory form of self-injurious behaviour directly to the cause of the other disabilities inherent in the Lesch-Nyhan syndrome (Nyhan, 1972).

One of the most important features of this approach is its capacity to indicate the likely strength of environmental contributions to behaviours identified (Billings et al, 1992;  Rutter et al, 1990).    For, whenever a behaviour is identified as being present in a proportion of people but not universally among those who are affected with a given condition, then there is the need to consider other aetiologies of behaviour.

A good example is the peculiar skin picking of Prader-Willi syndrome. This behaviour is common in Prader-Willi subjects, but not universally-so (Clarke et al, 1989). Most importantly in all of these situations, there is the need to consider some environmental contribution (Plomin, 1991).

One attraction of the genomic approach is therefore its capacity to identify the actual mathematical strength of the genetic influence on behaviour, and so in turn to indicate how much of the variance might be due to environmental factors.

**Phenomic** In the phenomic approach to behavioural phenotypes, we begin with observations of the behavioural phenotype per se.    It works this way. A group of individuals is observed to have certain behavioural characteristics in common.    The behavioural profile may be unusual, but as yet it is not known to be due to any identifiable biological condition. However there is good reason to group them together as they have common features, such as only occurring in one sex, or the recognition of a common predictable natural history.

A good example of a disorder which has been identified by the phenomic approach is Rett Syndrome. This condition is characterised by midline repetitive hand movements, with onset early in life. There is an idiosyncratic pattern of an evolution of changing symptoms over time, with a period of autistic type regression in early childhood, followed by the re-emergence of the capacity for social learning later. Throughout childhood into adult life, there is increasing muscle tone, resulting in an eventual picture of a flexed posture with generalised spastic paresis and mental retardation (Hagberg, 1985). It is most striking that only live females have as yet been described with this condition. This strongly suggests that the disorder has a genetic basis (Kerr, 1992).

Another notable examples of this approach has been Prader- Willi syndrome. This syndrome has been recognised for many years as a separate condition, equally common in males and females. It is characterised by a particular pattern of insatiable carbohydrate over-eating, and includes hypogonadism and tissue laxity. A gene for this condition has been identified on chromosome 15: a deletion at the 15q site (Butler et al 1986). Currently, the proportion of individuals is rising who on clinical phenomic diagnosis have Prader-Willi syndrome are found to have this gene. Moreover, there are more recent reports of mood disorders and anxiety regulation problems in Prader-Willi syndrome (Whitman and Accardo, 1987; Whitman and Greenswag, 1991). The presence of such socially crippling difficulties is important to note in planning care for affected individuals.

These are two notable examples of the phenomic approach, which starts with description of a phenotype including behavioural observations in the study of syndromes associated with mental retardation. In different ways, the study of these two disorders illustrate the strength of the phenomic approach. In the case of Prader-Willi syndrome, a gene has now been identified. In the case of Rett syndrome, the identification of a biological cause is still awaited, but is made possible because of the available descriptions of the behavioural phenotype. In both cases, meticulous behavioural observation has been crucial in the initial delineation of the syndrome. This has in turn paved the way for investigation of aetiology and pathogenesis to proceed.

## *Behavioural Measurement*

In detecting and measuring behavioural phenotypes, it is necessary to decide in advance just what is to be measured. For example, in some cases it may be appropriate to concentrate on just a few behaviours, or even on one type of behaviour. This will generally be in those cases where there is already good evidence of specific behavioural anomalies occurring in some condition(s). More often, a more general assessment of behaviour is required, for there are so many biological disorders in which there is as yet little behavioural information. Here, it may be useful to give some consideration to the four principal elements of behaviour we encounter in behavioural phenotypes - cognition, language, motor, social - as detailed in the definition of behavioural phenotype above.

Information on developmental attainments is also of great value, and often indispensable. This is because any set of behaviours might be a reflection of the individual's general developmental level, or might be occurring in relation to some specific developmental delay, for example of language function.

### Questionnaires

The informant-based questionnaire has probably been the most widely-used type of instrument for the investigation of behavioural phenotypes. As a research approach, the use of such a tool has many advantages. Firstly, and most importantly for practical purposes, there are the issues of ease of administration and the possibility of accessing large samples. The latter issue refers to the use of questionnaires distributed through such special interest forums as clinics with a special interest in certain disorders, and particularly family/syndrome support societies. Also, there are various means by which these questionnaires can be used: for example, by post as an adjunct to an interview or clinical examination or through distribution at large group meetings. It should be noted, incidentally, that the latter method seems to be favoured by many syndrome support societies.

Two informant questionnaires are worthy of special mention. These are the Developmentally-Delayed Version of the Child Behaviour Checklist (DD-CBC) and the SSBP Postal Questionnaire. To date, these two have been most widely employed in studies on behavioural phenotypes.

The DD-CBC has the advantage of being a derivative of one of the most successful tools used in child psychiatric diagnostic research, the original Achenbach CBC (McConachy and Achenbach, 1988). Indeed, several studies of behavioural phenotypes have successfully employed the latter instrument, rather than its adaptation for developmentally delayed subjects (e.g. Wood et al 1995). The DD-CBC was piloted on a very large population of developmentally delayed individuals (Einfeld and Tonge, 1991). This is a particularly useful feature, in that there is therefore useful control data. The authors have proposed that this questionnaire might be of considerable value in behavioural phenotypes research.

The other questionnaire recommended for work in this area - SSBP postal questionnaire - is an instrument which has been designed specifically to be sensitive to cross-syndrome differences in behavioural phenotypes. The SSBP PQ includes developmental information, and is primarily intended for use with children (aged 2 to 18 years) (O'Brien, 1994). An adult version of the scale has now been piloted (O'Brien, 1996).

### Interview Schedules

Interview schedules are particularly useful tools for the assessment of behavioural phenotypes. The adoption of an interview schedule is more likely to lead to greater validity than when a questionnaire is employed. This is most apparent where a trained skilled interviewer is able to use the interview situation to clarify and explain the meaning of the question items for the interviewee, and also to ensure that (s)he has correctly understood and recorded the responses given by the informant. In short, it is the task of the interviewer to keep in tune with the interviewee.

Furthermore, in the case of interviews concerning behaviour, examples of recent behaviours can be discussed in detail. In other words, the whole emphasis is to relate the interview, via the informant's observations of behaviour, as closely as possible to the subject's manifest behaviour.

Certain interview schedules have already proven to be particularly promising in the assessment and measurement of behavioural phenotypes.

The Handicap Behaviour and Skills Schedule (Wing, 1980) is a useful semi-structured informant based interview, which takes between 50 and 90 minutes to complete by a trained interviewer, preferably one who is a qualified clinician. The informant should be a parent or carer who knows the subject well. It is also recommended that the subject should be at least briefly observed as part of the interview examination.

Much of the material in the schedule is skills-based, including social skills. Approximately half of the items relate to autistic-type behaviours and related cognitive deficits. The instrument yields a single score, derived from the Vineland Scale. It has been used in individuals with all levels of intellectual and developmental disability. Supplementary question items are available for testing of very mildly retarded individuals.

The Present Behaviour Examination-Mental Handicap Version (O'Brien and Whitehouse, 1990) is a pre-coded forced choice informant-based interview, which takes around 90 minutes to complete. Informants should be any carer who can supply details of behaviour over the twenty-four hour period, i.e. including sleep-related behaviour. The approach taken in this interview has been the basis of a new instrument - the Behavioural Phenotypes Interview (Elsawi et al 1996). This interview schedule has the advantage of having been designed and developed for the specific purpose of the study of behavioural phenotypes.

The Autism Diagnostic Interview (Le Couteur et al 1989) is a highly-specialised interview schedule for the diagnostic assessment of autism and related pervasive developmental disorders. It is without doubt the one instrument for this purpose which is of the highest pedigree, with unrivalled sensitivity and specificity in measurement. Researchers interested in its use must contact the authors and arrange to attend a special training course to learn techniques of its administration. Notably, a shorter version of this tool is now available, which is of particular value to the busy clinician.

## Behavioural Phenotypes of Important Congenital Conditions

In the descriptions of individual conditions which follows, the genetic basis of each condition is briefly outlined along with some of the more important physical findings. This is followed by recent findings of behavioural and psychological phenotypes. The emphasis throughout is to demonstrate the clinical importance of such findings, particularly in respect of individualised holistic case management planning.

### Aicardi Syndrome

An X-linked dominant disorder which manifests only in girls as it is lethal in males conceptuses Diagnosis relies on agenesis of corpus callosum, severe epilepsy (infantile spasms / hypsarrhythmia), and typical choroidoretinal lacunae - unusual lesions found in the eye. Commonly results in severe disability, lethargy, self-injury, aggression and frequent night wakening (O'Brien, 1994).

### Angelman Syndrome

A mostly sporadic, non-familial congenital disorder of severe learning disability/mental retardation, which features inappropriate bouts of laughter and a jerky, ataxic pattern of movement and gait. Much recent work has focussed on the characteristically cheerful and excitable temperament most individuals display - also on expressive language delay and deviance, in the context of comparatively preserved receptive skills (Clayton-Smith, 1993).

## Cornelia de Lange Syndrome

A rare disorder (estimated around 1 in 40,000 to 100,000), which is also known as Amsterdam Dwarfism. The cause is unknown and the condition is not usually familial. There is a typical facial appearance with a small upturned nose, anteverted nostrils, neat well-defined eyebrows which fan out laterally as well as meeting together. With age, the eyebrows typically become bushy, and the nose and lips prominent. Psychological research has concentrated on language function, including guttural tone, the occurrence of autistic-type features, and of self-stimulatory behaviour, often of a self-injurious nature (Ireland et al, 1993).

## Down Syndrome

The commonest single genetic syndromal cause of learning disability, with an overall occurrence on 1 in 600 live births, being increasingly common with increasing maternal age, ranging from 1 in 2500 at maternal age under 30 years, rising to 1 in 32 at maternal age over 45 years. Three genetic sub-types of this trisomy (21) syndrome are recognised:

- 95% are non-familial, sporadic 47XX cases arising from non-disjunction (a "mishap" at one stage of cell division.). The recurrence risk following one case of this type in a family is 1 in 200.
- Up to 5% are translocations, where an exchange of the obligate region (the crucial piece of chromosomal material of which an extra piece is required to manifest the Down Syndrome) occurs between, usually, chromosomes 14 and 21. Some cases of this type are familial. The recurrence risk is 1 in 4, or higher.
- 1-2% are mosaics, where both trisomy 21 and normal cell lines occur in the same individual. This usually results in a lesser degree of intellectual disability.

This familiar condition has been much-studied, especially concerning the occurrence of Alzheimer-type dementia in middle aged and elderly subjects, reported by some to be as common as 50% of those aged 40 years or over (Collacott, 1993). Other research has concentrated on the apparently high prevalence of hyperactivity in boys with Down Syndrome, the comparatively infrequent occurrence of autism (given the level of learning disability/mental retardation which occurs in the syndrome) and the relationship between visual acuity problems and difficulties in the area of empathy and emotional understanding which have been reported.

## Fragile X Syndrome

Fragile X-Syndrome is an X-linked condition, but one which does not conform to the classical genetic pattern of expression of X-linked recessive conditions, which affect only males while being transmitted by carrier females. In Fragile X-Syndrome, women are also affected, albeit to a lesser extent.

The principal gene involved in the syndrome (designated FMR-1) is at the tip of the X-chromosome, but similar genes have also been identified at other sites: the significance of these other genes is as yet uncertain. The physical features of the condition are variable, classically large, prominent or poorly-folded ears, long face, and post-pubertal testicular enlargement in the majority of men. Intelligence is typically in the mild learning disability / mental retardation range.

The behavioural phenotype is striking, with social anxiety and gaze avoidance, a characteristic language disorder, stereotypic movements and poor concentration. All of these features, including the degree of intellectual disability, are more pronounced in affected males than females (Turk, 1992).

## Lesch-Nyhan Syndrome

An X-linked recessive disorder, involving a deficiency of an enzyme involved in purine metabolism (hypoxanthine phosphoribosyl transferase). Severe retardation occurs, with death in early adulthood being usual. Self-injurious behaviour is a prominent and severe feature: this has long been known to be uncontrollable, but unwelcome by affected individuals, who will cooperate with efforts made to prevent them injuring themselves, even including the controversial use of physical restraints - employed in some cases where severe self-mutilation has occurred (Nyhan, 1976).

## Noonan Syndrome

Noonan Syndrome is an autosomnal dominant condition, variable both in its penetrance (occurrence) and expressivity (severity). The variability of these two is of such an extent that many cases are very mild, and probably go unrecognised. It is quite common, probably around 1 in 1000 live births.

Physical features usually comprise short stature, a characteristic appearance (the combination of the latter two is often likened to Turner

Syndrome), and certain congenital heart defects; notable narrowing of the pulmonary valve. Studies of Noonan Syndrome have reported stubborn, repetitive behaviour, and poor socialisation, in the context of low normal or mildly retarded IQ: only around 2/3 have intellectual disability of such a degree as constitutes mental retardation (Sharland et al 1992).

## Phenylketonuria

This autosomnal recessive disorder of metabolism (of phenylalanine: the enzyme involved is phenylalanine hydroxylase) has an overall incidence of around 1 in 10,000 live births. Most cases are detected early in life through routine screening programmes, with the implementation of treatment by special diet, low in phenylalanine, which aims to prevent build up of the latter to brain-damaging levels. Even so, intellectual and behavioural difficulties are common in treated cases. Such individuals often have poor concentration, dis-inhibition, irritability, anxiety and socialisation problems (Medical Research Council, 1993).

## Prader-Willi Syndrome

Prader-Wili Syndrome is usually sporadic, not familial. The genetic basis of the condition is complicated, and not yet fully understood. The same gene (on Chromosome 15, at the site 15q 11-13) is implicated in Angelman Syndrome, but in Prader-Willi Syndrome it is of paternal origin, whereas it comes from the mother's genes in Angelman Syndrome. (There are some technical exceptions, when there is uni-parental disomy of chromosome 15 - the origin is then maternal for Prader-Willi, paternal for Angelman: the principal is the same; parental source affects ultimate gene expression.)

The most pronounced physical features of the Prader-Will phenotype are largely determined by the behavioural phenotype, with its insatiable carbohydrate over-eating, in addition to the other behavioural problems outlined earlier in this chapter (Curfs and Fryns, 1992).

## Rett Syndrome

A disorder of uncertain cause, Rett Syndrome is presumed to be genetic, given its unique occurrence in females. It is thought that a gene mutation occurs on the X-chromosome, and, being dominant, is lethal to males but progressively damaging to females. The longitudinal changes in the disorder are summarised earlier in this chapter (Hagberg, 1993).

### Smith-Magenis Syndrome

This is a rare condition, incidence probably around 1 in 50,000 live births. There is a variable physical phenotype, most notably a "cupid Bow" shape to the upper lip, broad face and nasal bridge, flat mid-face and a deep hoarse voice. Learning difficulties are also variable, from mild to severe mental retardation, most probably in the moderate band. Behaviour, however, is florid and dramatic, with a picture of self-injury which typically includes head-banging, wrist and hand biting, and even pulling out finger and toe nails. Sensitivity to pain is thought to be impaired (Greenberg et al, 1991).

### Sotos Syndrome

A sporadic, non-familial, condition, sometimes called cerebral gigantism. Prevalence unknown, because the features are so variable in expression. Typically presents with large body size, accelerated growth, advanced bone age, and a characteristic facial appearance with high forehead, prominent jaw, premature eruption of teeth and sparseness of hair, in addition to other eye and nasal findings. The main behavioural problems are in the area of aggression and emotional immaturity: given the large stature and appearance of the subjects, these problems assume greater importance (Rutter and Cole, 1991).

### Tuberous Sclerosis

Tuberous Sclerosis (TS) is an autosomnal dominant with variable expression; there is also a high incidence of new mutations. The condition is not uncommon, with a prevalence of approximately 1 in 7000. The condition has a classic triad of epilepsy, learning disability / mental retardation and certain skin problems - notably the so-called "adenoma sebaceum" rash. In fact many individuals only display the latter pathognomonic vascular malformations on the face: properly described as facial angiofibromata.

IQ varies enormously, according to brain involvement of blood vessel malformations - essentially the same as those which appear on the face, although referred to in the brain as hamartomata - from severe retardation to normal intelligence. The most prominent psychological findings are of generally disturbed, distractable and disinhibited behaviour, often amounting to an autistic / hyperactive constellation. This may be closely related to brain pathology, and often proves difficult to treat. Drug therapy is of limited success. The present author prefers the use of anti-epileptic drugs such as carbamazepine for this purpose (Hunt and Dennis, 1987).

### Williams Syndrome

Also often called Idiopathic infantile hypercalcaemia, Williams Syndrome is a fairly uncommon condition with an incidence of around 1 in 20,000 live births. Most cases are sporadic. The genetic basis of the disorder is a gene (microdeletion on chromosome 7: 7q11.23) which disrupts the production of elastin, an important constituent of the body's connective tissue. Consequently, there are problems in the heart and arterial walls of affected people.

IQ is often in the moderate / severe mental retardation range, (more than 50% cases) 40% mild and around 5% borderline / low average. Most individuals therefore require special schooling as children.

Physical health screening is also clearly a major issue for this multi-system disorder.

The behavioural phenotype typically comprises: poor peer relations; outgoing, socially disinhibited reactions to others; excessively inappropriate affection towards adults (in affected children) good expressive language, with an odd character sometimes referred to as "cocktail party" language. Hyperaccusis, hypersensitivity to sound, in almost universal.

It is also suggested that a capacity to over-empathise with the feelings of others is common, to an extent which can be quite emotionally disabling, resulting in extreme emotional upsets: quite at odds with the "easy going" image people with Willams Syndrome tend to give on first impressions (Udwin and Yule, 1990).

## *Conclusions*

Detection of behavioural phenotypes is important and beneficial for the individuals concerned. Only by such a holistic and thorough evaluation of people affected by genetically-determined conditions, can properly informed casework proceed optimally. There are inherent problems in the area of 'labelling' and setting up false expectations but these should be met with a spirit of realistic appraisal and thorough assessment of each case. In this way, any behavioural phenotype 'label' will be an enabling one, especially for case planning and service provision.

# References

Billings, B. P.R., Beckworth, J. & Alper, J. S., (1992). The genetic analysis of human behaviour: a new era? *Social Science and Medicine.* 35 (3): 227-38.

Butler, M.G., Meaney, F.J. & Palmer, C.G. (1986) Clinical and cytogenetic survey of 39 individuals with Prader-Labhart-Willi syndrome. *American Journal of Medical Genetics*, 23, 793-809.

Clarke, D. J., Waters, J. & Corbett, J. A. (1989). Adults with Prader-Willi syndrome: abnormalities of sleep and behaviour. *Journal of the Royal Society of Medicine,* 82, 21-24.

Clayton-Smith, J. (1993) Clinical research on Angelman Syndrome in the UK: observations on 82 affected individuals. *American Journal of Medical Genetics*, 46, 12-15.

Collacott, R. (1993) Epilepsy, dementia and adaptive behaviour in Down syndrome. *Journal of Intellectual Disability Research*, 37, 153-160.

Curfs, L.M.G. & Fryns, J.P. (1992) Prader-Willi Syndrome: a review with special attention to the cognitive and behavioural profile. *Birth Defects: Original Articles Series,* 28, 99-104.

Elsawi, M., Bax, M. O'Brien, G. & Yule, W. (1996) Validity study of syndromal behavioural phenotypes. Genetic Counselling, 7, 2, 164.

Flint, J. and Yule, W. (1993). Behavioural Phenotypes. In M. Rutter & L. Hersov, (eds.) *Recent Advances in Child and Adolescent Psychiatry, 3^{rd} Edition.* Oxford: Blackwell Scientific.

Greenberg, F., Guzzetta, V., Montes de Oca-Luna, R. Magenis, R.E., Smith, A.C.M., Richter, S.F., Kondo, I., Dobyns, W.B., Patel, P.I.& Lupski, J.R. (1991). Molecular analysis of the Smith-Magenis Syndrome: A possible contiguous gene associated with del(17)(p11.2p11.2) in nine patients. *American Journal of Medical Genetics*, 24, 393-414.

Hagberg, B. (1985) Rett Syndrome, prevalence and impact on progressive severe mental retardation in girls. *Acta Paediatrica Scandinavica*, 74, 405-408.

Hagberg, B. (ed.) (1993) Rett Syndrome: a comprehensive review of the literature. *Clinics in Developmental Medicine no. 127*, London: Mac Keith Press.

Hunt, A. and Dennis, J. (1987) Psychiatric disorder among children with tuberous sclerosis. *Developmental Medicine and Child Neurology*, 29, 190-198.

Ireland, M., Donnai, D. & Burn, J. (1993) Brachman-de Lange Syndrome. Delineation of the clinical phenotype. *American Journal of Medical Genetics,* 47, 959-964.

Kerr, A. (1992) Rett Syndrome: British Longitudinal Study (1982-1990) and 1990 Survey. In J.J. Roosendall (ed.) *Mental Retardation and Medical Care, April 21-24, 1991.* Publisher: Uitgeverij Kerckbosch, Zeist.

Le Couteur, A., Rutter, M., Lord, C., Rios, P., Robertson, S., Holdgrafer, M. & McLennan, J. (1989) Autism diagnostic interview: a standardised investigator-based instrument. *Journal of Autism and Developmental Disorders,* 19, 363-387.

McConachy, S.H. & Achenbach, T.M. (1988) *Practical Guide for the Child Behaviour Checklist and Related Materials.* Burlington, VT: University of Vermont Department of Psychiatry.

Medical Research Council Working Party on Phenylketonuria (1993) Phenylketonuria due to phenylalanine hydroxylase deficiency: an unfolding story. *British Medical Journal,* 306, 115-119.

Nyhan, W. L. (1972). Behavioural phenotypes in organic genetic disease. Presidential address to the Society for Paediatric Research, 1 May, 1971, *Paediatric Research,* 6, 1-9.

Nyhan, W. L. (1976) Behaviour in Lesch-Nyhan Syndrome. *Journal of Autism and Childhood Schizophrenia,* 6, 255-252.

O'Brien, G. & Whitehouse, A. (1990) A Psychiatric Study of Deviant Eating Behaviour among Mentally Handicapped Adults. *British Journal of Psychiatry,* 157, 281-284.

O'Brien, G. (1994) The Behavioural and Developmental Consequences of Corpus Callosal Agenesis and Aicardi Syndrome. In M. Lassonde & M.A. Jeeves (eds.) *Callosal Agenesis - The Natural Split Brain,* Plenum Press, New York.

O'Brien, G. (1996) A Comparative study of young children and adults with Fragile X syndrome. *Genetic Counseling,* 7, 2, 167.

Plomin, R. (1991). Behavioural genetics. In P. R. McGugh & V. A. McCusick, (eds.) *Genes, Brain and Behaviour: Research publications - Association for Research in Nervous and Mental Diseases.* 69: 165-80.

Rutter, M., Bolton, P., Harrington, R., Le Couteur, A. L., MacDonald, H. & Simonoffe, E. (1990a), Genetic factors and child psychiatric disorders - A review of research strategies. *Journal of Child Psychology and Psychiatry,* 31, 1, 3-37.

Sharland, M., Burch, M., McKenna, W.M., Paton, M.A. (1992) A clinical study of Noonan Syndrome. *Archives of Disease in Childhood,* 67, 178-183.

Turk, J. (1992) Fragile X Syndrome - on the way to a behavioural phenotype. *British Journal of Psychiatry,* 160, 24-35.

Udwin, O. & Yule, W. (1990) A cognitive and behavioural phenotype in Williams Syndrome. *Journal of Clinical and Experimental Neuropsychology,* 32, 129-141.

Whitman, B.Y. & Accardo, P. (1987) Emotional symptoms in Prader-Willi syndrome adolescents. *American Journal of Medical Genetics,* 28, 897-905.

Whitman, B.Y. & Greenswag, L.R. (1991) The use of mood and behaviour altering drugs in persons with Prader-Willi Syndrome. *Paediatric Research,* 29,

Wing, L. (1980) The Medical Research Council Handicap Behaviour and Skills (HBS) Schedule. In E. Strong, S.T.R. Ongren, A. Dupont & J.A. Nielsen (eds.) Epidemiological Research as Basis for the Organisation of Extramural Psychiatry. *Acta Psychiatrica Scandinavica,* 62 (supplement 285) 241-247.

Wood, A., Massarano, A., Super, M. & Harrington, R. (1995) Behavioural aspects and psychiatric findings in Noonan's syndrome. *Archives of Diseases in Childhood,* 72, 153-155.

**Gregory O'Brien** is Consultant Psychiatrist in Learning Disabilities at Northgate Hospital and Senior Lecturer in the University Department of Psychiatry at Newcastle-upon-Tyne. His interests include the study of behavioural phenotypes, psychiatric sequelae of child head injury and the adult outcome of child disabilities and related pervasive developmental disorders.

**Contact Address**
Northgate Hospital
Morpeth
Northumberland , NE61 3BP
England

# 13
# *Advances in the Assessment of Behaviour: The Role of Brain Imaging*

## Dene Robertson and Declan Murphy

Recently developed *in vivo* neuroimaging techniques enable detailed examination of the structure and function of human brain, and have particular applications to people with a learning disability. It is not our intention to provide an exhaustive overview of all brain imaging studies in people with learning disability. Rather, we will review the brain imaging techniques which are currently available. We will:

1 Show how they are being used to understand normal brain development,
2 Explain how they can be used to study the biological determinants of brain development, using Turner's Syndrome as an example,
3 Illustrate research findings in three groups of people in whom learning disability occurs: those with Fragile-X Syndrome, Autism, and Down's Syndrome,
4 Discuss the potential clinical applications of *in vivo* brain imaging in people with Huntingdon's Disease and epilepsy ,
5 Suggest ways in which *in vivo* neuroimaging techniques should modify clinical practice in people with a learning disability.

We hope that, by the end of this chapter, the reader will appreciate how modern neuroimaging techniques can be used to understand brain structure and function in health and disease.

## *Neuroimaging Techniques*

Structural techniques (computerised tomography and magnetic resonance imaging) allow the qualitiative and quantitative examination of brain anatomy, whereas functional techniques (positron emission tomography, single photon emission tomography, magnetic resonance spectroscopy, and functional magnetic resonance imaging) enable us to study how the brain works. In practice, structural and functional techniques provide a fuller picture when used together.

## Structural Brain Imaging

***Computerised Tomography (CT) Scanning***    It relies on the acquisition of X-ray images, which are reconstructed by computer to provide a slice by slice representation of the brain. The resulting image, however, provides a level of detail that is inferior to that obtained with MRI. Also, CT is less good at visualizing some brain areas (e.g. the inferior temporal lobes), and it exposes the patient to ionizing radiation.

***Magnetic Resonance Imaging (MRI)***    MRI provides more detailed images than CT (e.g. better differentiation between grey and white matter), and does not expose the patient to ionizing radiation. MRI works by detecting the relative amounts of common atomic nuclei in tissue. Computers are used to reconstruct the information that has been received, producing an image. These images can then be 'read' by a neuroradiologist, to give a qualitative interpretation of the data.

In contrast, quantitative investigation involves objective measurement. Quantitative investigations are especially useful because results can be directly compared to known neuroanatomical 'norms' and to other study results. Also, many differences between normal and abnormal brain development are subtle, and may go unobserved if images are analysed qualitatively.

The strength of the magnetic field causes many metals to move around if placed in the scanner, and unwanted electric currents may be induced in vital equipment. For these reasons, some people may not be scanned using MRI (e.g. those with cerebral artery aneurysm clips, cardiac pacemakers, and cochlear implants).

## Functional Brain Imaging

***Magnetic Resonance Spectroscopy (MRS)***    The principles behind MRS are the same as those that underlie MRI. Within prescribed regions of interest within brain, the relative abundancies of different biomolecules are calculated. MRS allows the *in vivo* estimation of neuronal density, membrane turnover, and neuronal metabolic activity.

***Functional magnetic resonance imaging (fMRI)***    fMRI is a new technique that provdes the highest level of spatial detail of the functional techniques described here. The basic principles are as for MRI. Regions of brain which are activated during cognitive tasks are detected by comparing the signals from off (inactive) and on (active) phases of an activation paradigm. Patterns of activation in response to the cognitive demands of the task are mapped onto standard MR images, revealing the location of the neural substrate for the task.

***Positron emission tomography (PET)*** In PET, radioactive tracer compounds are administered and become distributed within the brain. When atoms contained within these radiotracers decay, the photons 'given off' are detected by equipment surrounding the subject's head. Computers are used to calculate the distribution of the tracer. The resulting images are often mapped onto a precise anatomical image (e.g. from MRI), to enable brain function to be related to brain anatomy. PET techniques can be used to study the brain in health and disease, assess disease progression, and measure response to treatment interventions.

***Single photon emission tomography (SPET)*** Like PET, SPET also relies on the administration of radio-pharmaceuticals and their distribution within brain. The principles of data acquisition are similar to those of PET. In comparison to PET, image detail is generally inferior, but it is much cheaper and therefore more widely available.

## Normal Brain Development and Ageing

We need to understand healthy brain development and ageing in order to understand how this differs in people with a learning disability. Brain development and ageing have been studied using both structural and functional neuroimaging techniques.

Human brain tissue is principally composed of grey matter and white matter. Grey matter contains the nerve cell bodies and forms the cerebral cortex (outer lining of the brain). It is also found deep within the cerebral hemispheres in structures known collectively as the subcortical nuclei. These include the caudate, lentiform (composed of globus pallidus and putamen) and thalamic nuclei - one of which is found in each cerebral hemisphere. These subcortical structures are buried in white matter which is composed mainly of the myelinated axons of nerve cells - myelin is a fatty substance vital for electrical conduction by some nerve cells. Large bundles of myelinated axons make up the white matter tracts which are responsible for the connections between widely separated brain regions. Within the cerebral hemispheres there are also ventricles (cavities) which are filled with cerebrospinal fluid (CSF).

There is no sudden transition from development to ageing in human brain. These processes are continuous, and occur at different rates within different brain regions. During childhood brain weight increases dramatically. By the age of ten years, it is four times its weight at birth, but thereafter gradually declines (Debakan and Sadowsky, 1978). MRI studies have reported that white matter tracts can be identified at one year of age, and that these continue to develop into adolescence. The total white matter volume peaks at about 20 years of age, and then remains stable (e.g. Barkowich *et al.*, 1988; Christophe *et al.*, 1990). However, the total amount of grey matter relative to the total amount of white matter is greatest at around 4 years of age, and decreases throughout adulthood, suggesting that grey matter atrophy is responsible for the age-related decrease in brain volume. Post mortem and CT findings are in agreement with these MRI results (e.g. DeLeo *et al.*, 1985). Quantitative MRI studies have also examined age-related loss of brain matter on a region by region basis, and indicate that the ageing process effects some brain regions (e.g. the frontal lobes) more than others (e.g. the temporal lobes) (DeCarli *et al.*, 1994; Murphy *et al.*, 1992).

Age-related changes in brain structure also vary according to sex. This is of particular interest because gender differences in brain ageing may underlie gender differences in neuropsychiatric disorder. For example, CT studies report that the ventricles begin to increase in volume (implying grey matter loss) in the fifth decade in men and the sixth in women (e.g. Kaye *et al.*, 1992). However, atrophy occurs more rapidly in women once it has started (Takeda and Matsuzawa, 1985). MRI studies of sex differences in brain ageing are in disagreement. Although some find no sex difference (e.g.Coffey *et al.*, 1992), others (e.g. Cowell *et al.*, 1994) report that males have a greater age-related loss of whole brain volume than females, and that age-related atrophy is asymmetric in males but not in females. One MRI study has investigated the effects of sex differences on regional brain volumes. Murphy *et al.* (1996) reported that age-related loss of brain tissue was significantly greater in males than females in whole brain, frontal and temporal lobes, whereas it was greater in females than males in hippocampus and parietal lobes. These results strongly suggest a role for the sex chromosomes and/or gonadal hormones in the development and ageing of healthy brain.

Functional neuroimaging techniques have also been used to examine brain development and ageing. For instance, when PET was used to examine the cerebral metabolic rates of children from 5 days to 15 years (Chugani *et al.*, 1987), cerebral metabolism was found to have decreased by 50% in those aged over 9 years. Also, a SPET study reported that maximal brain metabolism occurred at about 5 years (Chiron *et al.*, 1992). Because most brain energy expenditure is due to the function of synaptic connections between cells, these results suggest that there is a large decrease in synaptic density as childhood progresses.

Using PET and FDG, Murphy *et al.* (1996) reported age-related decreases in resting glucose metabolism also occur during adulthood. Brain regions most affected included the temporal and parietal lobes, thalamus and hippocampus. Moreover, these changes vary according to sex. For example, age-related decline in brain metabolism is asymmetric in males, but symmetric in females, and women have significant age-related decreases in hippocampal glucose metabolism but men do not. These gender differences in brain ageing occur in regions which are essential to cognitive function and are implicated in neuropsychiatric disease. They may therefore underlie gender differences in the prevalence and symptomatology of age-related disorders such as late-onset schizophrenia and Alzheimer's disease.

Using PET, it is also possible to examine how different regions of brain are functionally connected. For example, if activity in one brain region depends on activity in another, a change in metabolism in one will be related to change in metabolism in the other. Thus, Horwitz *et al.* (1986) studied the functional relationships between brain areas in young and old subjects, and reported significant age-related decreases in functional connectivity between frontal and parietal areas, and between the left and right parietal lobes. They hypothesized that these age-related changes are associated with some of the neuropsychological deficits seen in the elderly, for example those that depend heavily on the integrated function of anterior and posterior brain regions (such as tasks of attention).

Many cognitive functions are lateralised to one cerebral hemisphere, and PET studies suggest that lateralization is maintained during healthy ageing. For example, when subjects performed recognition tasks for words and faces (Berardi *et al.*, 1990), subjects with a better verbal memory performance had greater left than right parietal metabolism, and those with a better memory for faces had greater right than left parietal metabolism. However, a PET cognitive activation study reported that when healthy subjects were required to encode and then recognise faces, young subjects showed increased activity in the right hemisphere, but elderly subjects did not (Grady *et al.*, 1995) - suggesting that decreased right hemisphere function and defective encoding may be responsible for age-related deficits in memory for faces.

In summary, we need to study how healthy brain develops and ages before we can understand how this process differs in people with a learning disability. Gender differences in the structure and function of healthy brain suggest that sex steroids and sex chromosomes have a crucial part to play in brain development and ageing. Also, age-related gender differences in brain structure and function may explain age-related changes in cognition and neuropsychiatric disorders.

## Turner's Syndrome as a Model for Examining Brain Development

Evidence of the importance of the X-chromosome in brain development comes from neuropsychological studies of people who possess abnormal numbers of X chromosomes. For example, girls who are 47,XXX have delayed language development (e.g. Pennington *et al.*, 1980), and 49,XXXXY males have better visuospatial than verbal skills (e.g. Curfs *et al.*, 1990).

Women with Turner's Syndrome (TS, 45X) have better verbal than visuospatial skills and abnormalities of social interaction (Murphy *et al.*, 1993). Because TS females lack one/part of one X chromosome and sex steroids, they allow us to investigate the effects of the X chromosome and sex steroids on brain and behaviour. A quantitative MRI study of females with TS reported significant bilateral decreases in the volume of hippocampus, parieto-occipital brain matter, lenticular and thalamic nuclei compared to controls (46XX) (Murphy *et al*, 1993). Moreover, the cerebral hemispheres, caudate, and the lenticular and thalamic nuclei showed 'X chromosome dosage effects', indicating that these structures depend upon the X chromosome to develop normally. Hippocampal volume was decreased in the TS subjects, but did not show these effects, suggesting that hippocampal development depends to a greater degree on sex steroids.

Resting brain glucose metabolism has also been compared in TS females and controls, using FDG-PET. Clark *et al.* (1990) reported decreased metabolism in occipital and parietal cortices, and recently Murphy *et al.* (1997) reported that TS was associated with relative bilateral hypometabolism in association neocortices and insulae. In TS females there were also significant differences in cortical functional relationships originating bilaterally in the occipital cortices, and within the right hemisphere. Also, 'X chromosome dosage' effects existed in language ability and left middle temporal lobe metabolism, and in neuropsychological test scores and asymmetry of parietal metabolism, indicating that the X chromosome is involved in the function of the left and right association neocortices, and that in TS brain metabolic abnormalities are associated with cognitive deficits.

Thus, TS provides a model with which to study the effects of the X chromosome and sex steroids on brain and behaviour. The X chromosome and sex steroids appear to have differential effects on brain structure and function, and these may explain some of the neuropsychological and social deficits that are seen in TS.

## *Fragile X Syndrome (FRAX)*

FRAX is the commonest form of inherited learning disability, and is associated with a variable but decreased intellectual ability - from normal intelligence to severe learning disability - and behavioural abnormalities. FRAX is caused by an expansion of CGG triplet repeats (TRS) in the FMR-1 gene on the X chromosome. Healthy normal subjects have up to 50 TRS, premutation carriers of FRAX have 50-200 TRS, and people with the full FRAX mutation have more than 200 TRS (which causes loss of gene expression).

Although males and females with FRAX have similar cognitive and behavioural profiles, deficits tend to be more severe in males (e.g. Kemper *et al.*, 1986). Most males with the FRAX full mutation have mental retardation - usually in the moderate or severe range (Kemper *et al.*, 1988). In addition to an overall impairment of intelligence, people with FRAX have relatively greater deficits in some cognitive domains (e.g. attention, processing of sequential information, and short-term memory) compared to others (e.g. verbal abilities). Behavioural abnormalities include hyperactivity, stereotypies and social abnormalities which resemble those found in autism.

Qualitative CT studies in people with FRAX have reported mild ventricular dilatation or cerebral atrophy ( e.g. Rhoades, 1982; Veenema *et al.*, 1987). However, these findings were not replicated in a quantitative study (Schapiro *et al.*, 1995), which reported significantly increased intracranial volumes and right/left asymmetry of the lateral ventricles. Structural MRI studies have reported a significant decrease in volume of the cerebellar vermis and superior temporal gyri, and an increase in volume of the fourth ventricle and hippocampi in people with FRAX compared to controls (e.g. Reiss *et al.*, 1994). Moreover, in some cases the degree of structural abnormality was related to the % of active X chromosomes carrying the FRAX mutation (Reiss *et al.*, 1995). Also, a recent study reported that female premutation carriers of FRAX had increased hippocampal volumes compared to controls (Murphy *et al.*, 1996; in submission), suggesting that 'biological anticipation' occurs in premutation carriers of FRAX.

Thus, structural neuroimaging studies report that people with both the full FRAX mutation and premutation carriers have abnormalities in the development of brain regions involved in higher cognitive function.

FDG-PET has been used to investigate regional brain glucose metabolism in people with FRAX. Shapiro *et al.* (1995) reported that compared to controls, people with FRAX had significantly increased glucose metabolism in the cerebellar vermis, calcarine cortex and caudate nucleus. Also, people with FRAX had a significantly greater asymmetry of parietal lobe metabolism. Moreover, there were abnormalities of functional interaction between the left premotor region of cortex and the right lenticular nucleus which were similar in nature to those found in autism, suggesting that these may be responible for behavioural phenotypic similarities in FRAX and autistic individuals. Preliminary work using FDG-PET has examined female premutation carriers of FRAX (Murphy *et al.*, 1996; in submission). Compared to controls, female premutation carriers had relative increases in metabolism in hippocampus and cerebellum, and decreases in right sided cortical areas.

The abnormalities in brain structure and function in FRAX occur in brain regions which are involved in higher cognitive function and have high FMR-1 gene expression. They may therefore explain some of the deficits in cognitive ability that occur in people with FRAX. For example, the hippocampus is known to be involved in memory, and memory and hippocampal structure and function are abnormal in FRAX (Murphy *et al.*, 1996; Reiss *et al*,, 1995). In people with FRAX cognitive abilities are thought to decline in early adulthood, implying increased brain ageing. It has been reported that changes in the volumes of the hippocampi and superior temporal gyri are age-related (Reiss *et al.*, 1994), suggesting that age-related changes in cognitive ability may result from age-related changes in brain structure and function.

## *Autism*

Autism is characterised by severe deficits in language development, disturbance of social interaction, bizarre responses to the environment, and an onset at less than 30 months of age. Only 30% of people with autism have an IQ above 70, and 40% are severely or profoundly learning disabled. There are many reasons for believing that there is a biological basis to the disorder. For example, autism occurs more frequently in monozygotic than dizygotic twins, and in people with FRAX (approximately 5% of whom develop the disorder). Also, one third of people with autism develop epilepsy in adolescence. Not surprisingly, there has been much interest in the brain structure and function of people with autism.

Using CT, a number of investigators have reported abnormalities in ventricular size and in cerebral hemispheric asymmetry in people with autism (see: Lotspeich *et al.*, 1993, for a review). MRI studies have demonstrated widened parietal sulci (implying loss of parietal cortical grey matter)

(Courchesne *et al.*, 1993), and abnormalities in the area of posterior corpus callosum (Egaas *et al.*, 1995). These findings suggest that there may be a decrease in the number of axons connecting the parietal lobes, and a deficit in interhemispheric communication. Some MRI studies have reported cerebellar hypoplasia (e.g. Courchesne *et al.*, 1988; Gafney *et al.*, 1987), although this has not been replicated by others (e.g. Hashimoto *et al.*, 1993). There is, however, neuropsychological support for cerebellar abnormalities in autism, including increased latency in the extinction of the eye-blink response (Sears *et al.*, 1994), and evidence of abnormal motor development.

Studies of resting brain metabolism in autism are also in disagreement. SPET and FDG-PET, have reported brain metabolism as increased (e.g. de Volder *et al.*, 1987), decreased (e.g. Gillberg *et al.*, 1993), or unchanged (e.g. Zilbovicius *et al.*, 1992). However, studies which examined the functional relationships between different regions of brain reported that compared to controls, people with autism had significant differences in the metabolic relationship between frontal and parietal lobes and subcortical grey matter (Horwitz *et al.*, 1988), and a lack of metabolic asymmetry (Buchsbaum *et al.*, 1992). Also, a delay in the normal development of patterns of blood flow to the frontal cortex has also been reported in a study using SPET (Zilbovicius *et al.*, 1995). Because damage to the frontal lobes causes deficits in social interaction in people without autism, this suggests that social abnormalities in people with autism may be due to abnormal development of the frontal lobe function, and abnormalities in functional relationships between subcortical nuclei and association neocortex.

In summary, people with autism have generalised abnormalities in the development of brain structure and function. However, some brain areas may be more affected than others. Also, neural connectivity between brain regions is significantly affected, and this may explain the cognitive and social deficits seen people with autism.

## Down Syndrome (DS)

People with DS (trisomy 21) have a high prevalence of learning disability, and increased rates of age-related cognitive decline and Alzheimer's disease (Haxby, 1989). Also, there is evidence that people with DS have abnormalities in brain structure, neural integrity and metabolism.

A quantitative study of young adults with DS using CT reported that they had a reduced whole brain size (Shapiro *et al.*, 1989), which may be secondary to small stature. However, there is also CT evidence for abnormalities in brain morphometry, even when head size is taken into account. For example,

Pearlson *et al.* (1990) reported decreased temporal lobe volume in people with DS. A volumetric MRI study of people with Down's syndrome has reported morphomeric abnormalities in frontal cortex, cerebellum, parahippocampal gyrus and temporal cortex. (Kesslak *et al.*, 1994). Also, hippocampal area (even when corrected for head size) was significantly decreased, and was affected by ageing significantly more than in controls.

MRS studies of people with DS compared to controls reported no difference in brain NAA, creatine, or choline concentrations (Shonk and Ross, 1994), but did find a significant increase in the polyol sugar myoinositol (MI), which is also known to be increased in the CSF of DS subjects (Shetty *et al.*, 1995). Because the genes responsible for the passage of MI into cells are coded for on chromosome 21, and MI has significant effects on neural integrity and metabolism, abnormalities in MI metabolism may underlie some of the cognitive and behavioural deficits found in DS. However, these studies of MI were small, and did not examine brain areas involved in higher cognitive function. It is therefore unclear how increases in brain MI in people with DS are related to abnormalities in cognition, brain morphometry or neural integrity.

Studies of age-related differences in neural integrity in people with DS report increased choline concentration compared to controls (Murata *et al.*, 1993). Also, MRS studies of people without DS but with Alzheimer's disease (AD) reported abnormalities in choline (Meyerhoff *et al.*, 1992), NAA (e.g. Bruhn *et al.*, 1992), and myoinositol (Miller *et al.*, 1993). Thus, in people with DS, abnormalities in neuronal integrity and metabolism may be related to deficits in cognitive function, ageing, or AD. Further investigation is needed to tease apart the relative contributions of these factors in AD and DS.

## *Brain Imaging in Clinical Practice*

We have described the use of in vivo structural and functional techniques to investigate the biological determinants of brain structure and function in health and disease. We will now discuss two examples of neuropsychiatric disorders (Huntington's Disease and epilepsy) in which in vivo brain imaging has clinical applications, and then discuss how MRI may be used in the clinical practice of psychiatry for people with learning disability.

### Huntington's Disease (HD)

HD is an autosomoal dominant disorder with 100% penetrance and an average age of onset of 41 years. Patients with HD suffer from choreoathetosis (a movement disorder characterized by jerking and writhing movements which cease during sleep), a high prevalence of neuropsychiatric disorders (such as paranoid psychosis), and dementia. Recently, the cause of HD has been identified as an expansion of trinucleotide repeats (cf. FRAX, above) in IT15 (interesting transcript 15) located on the short arm of chromosome 4. People unaffected have six to 31 triplet repeats, whereas patients with HD have from 36 to 82 repeats. The role of the gene product, huntingtin, is unknown.

In addition to a 30% reduction in whole brain weight at post mortem, neuropathological studies report regional abnormalities, mainly in subcortical nuclei. These include gross abnormalities (in form and number) of spiny cells found in the caudate nuclei, significant loss of neurons from the putamen and to a lesser degree in the globus pallidus and prefrontal cortex.

In well established HD, both qualitative and quantitative structural neuroimaging studies (CT and MRI) consistently report decreased caudate nucleus size - for example, Sedvall et al. (1994) reported that the volumes of the caudate nuclei were reduced by as much as 50% in patients with mild to moderate functional impairment. Using CT, Starkstein et al. (1988) reported that reduction in 'bicaudate ratio' correlated with impairment on the Mini Mental State Exam (a measure of degree of dementia) - but not ratings of movement disorder - suggesting that anatomical abnormalities in caudate nuclei may underlie deficits in cognitive function. Also, using structural MRI, Harris et al. (1992) reported that decreased putaminal volume correlated with with neurological deficit but caudate volume did not, indicating that putaminal disease may be responsible for the movement disorder. This hypothesis is supported by results from SPET studies of blood flow, and PET studies of regional brain metabolism and dopamine (D1 and D2) receptor binding (Weeks et al., 1996) which reported that decreased tracer uptake in the caudate nucleus correlates mostly with overall intellectual function, whereas putaminal abnormalities correlate with degree of chorea. Animal models of HD reinforce these findings - bilateral lesions to the posterior putamen give rise to choreoathetosis closely resembling that found in HD (Burns et al., 1995).

Although it is now possible to identify people who will develop the classical symptoms of HD with genetic tests, clinical diagnosis of disease onset depends mainly on the early recognition of choreoathetosis. This may go unnoticed, or become confused with the understandable effects of anxiety. There is therefore a need for an objective diagnostic measure. The most promising avenues are measurement of putaminal and/or caudate volume using MRI, and regional cerebral blood flow and metabolism using SPET/PET. However, caudate atrophy is not always detected at disease onset, and in mild to moderate HD decrease in putaminal volume may exceed that of the caudate nucleus (Harris et al., 1992). Therefore, putaminal volume may be the most useful indicator of early disease. FDG-PET studies have reported decreased metabolism in the caudate nucleus and putamen which antedate the appearance of symptoms by several years. Thus, these may be a marker for presence of the HD gene and of little use in detecting disease onset. Findings with SPET differ little from those described for PET.

In summary, HD provides a model for the increasing clinical use of modern structural and functional neuroimaing techniques. Similar uses are likely to be found within the field of learning disability. For example, these techniques may be used to diagnose and monitor disease progression in neurodegenerative disorders such as Alzheimer's Disease and HD. Also, they may be used to assess response to interventions (including gene therapy) if these become available.

## Epilepsy

Epilepsy occurs in 1-2% of the general population, 18% of all learning disabled people, and 50% of those who are severely learning disabled. Seizures may be associated with syndromal learning disability (e.g. Lennox-Gestaut Syndrome or phenylketonuria), related to focal or diffuse brain damage, or idiopathic. Although the incidence of epilepsy generally decreases with age, epilepsy may develop later in life in people with autism, Down's syndrome and progressive neurodegenerative disorders (such as the lipidoses). Psychological disorders occur in about 30% of people with epilepsy, and 50% of those with epilepsy of temporal lobe origin. About one quarter of all cases become unresponsive to medication and lead to severe disability in adult life. Moreover, in a learning disabled population, epilepsy may increase the chance of institutional care. Therefore, epilepsy is associated with significant social, psychological, medical and financial consequences, and accurate diagnosis and management are essential.

Ninety percent of partial epilepsies - which constitute 60% of all epilepsy - have a temporal lobe origin, and give rise to complex partial (temporal lobe) seizures. The most common histopathologic finding in temporal lobe epilepsy is mesial temporal sclerosis (MTS) - a dense infiltration of hippocampus and amygdala with glial (non-neuronal) tissue, together with loss of neuronal cells - which is thought to arise from early cerebral insult (e.g. infantile febrile convulsions). Once MTS is present, seizures may lead to local chemical abnormalities, and further neuronal loss.

It is well established that surgical resection of the affected hippocampus/temporal lobe is effective in eliminating seizures or reducing seizure frequency in temporal lobe epilepsy which is refractory to medical treatment. However, prior to surgical intervention, it is vital to accurately identify the location of the epileptogenic focus, as well as functionally important brain structures to be avoided during surgery (e.g. those involved in memory, speech and movement). Although scalp electroencephalography (EEG) is often satisfactory for location of the seizure focus, invasive EEG techniques may be required. These include direct recording from the cortical surface with strip electrodes, and percutaneous recording from the temporal lobe itself.

It is likely that minimally invasive and non-invasive scanning techniques will make invasive EEG investigations less necessary. Because MRI has higher spatial resolution than CT, and increases the frequency with which epileptogenic foci are identified, structural MRI has rapidly outstripped CT in the presurgical evaluation of patients with temporal lobe epilepsy. Qualitiative T2 weighted coronal MR images are capable of identifying MTS (which has a high correlation with seizure origin in medial temporal structures), temporal lobe atrophy, mass lesions, and developmental lesions previously identified only after tissue resection. Quantitative MRI enables objective assessment of hippocampal volume, and increases the sensitivity of the technique. Thus, hippocampal volume may be compared to standard measurements of volume, or examined within the same patient by comparing the volumes of left and right hippocampi. There are high rates of concordance between abnormality detected on MRI, EEG, and post-surgical examination of resected tissue. Also, proton MRS has been used to examine in vivo regional neural integrity in humans with epilepsy and in animals. For example, when MR images of medial temporal lobe structures appear normal, MRS can detect alterations in the concentration of NAA and choline.

PET studies of regional cerebral metabolism and regional cerebral blood flow can be used to aid localisation of an epileptogenic focus when this is unclear from scalp EEG and/or MRI. PET reliably demonstrates hypoperfusion in the epileptogenic zone during the interictal period. Also, when SPET is used between seizures to study regional cerebral blood flow, regions of hypoperfusion correlate with areas of cortex within which epileptogenic foci are found. During seizures, SPET reveals local hyperperfusion superimposed on interictal hypoperfusion, and correctly identifies more epileptogenic foci than interictal testing. The reliability of SPET is further improved by comparison of ictal and interictal images in the same patient. Although PET is superior in resolution and yield to SPET, it is not possible to perform ictal studies with PET.

The assessment of language dominance is important in the pre-surgical evaluation of temporal lobe epilepsy, and language areas are avoided if possible during surgery. In a clinical setting, cerebral dominance for language is assessed using the Wada technique. This is an invasive procedure in which each hemisphere is selectively anaesthetised (by injection of sodium amytal into the external carotid artery), and resulting changes in linguistic performance are observed. Retention of linguistic function when the right hemisphere is anaesthetised indicates that the left hemisphere is dominant for language and vice versa. The Wada technique has an appreciable morbidity. However, simple cognitive activation tasks, (such as those involving verbal fluency) are known to activate classical language areas, and can be detected using PET, SPET or fMRI. As fMRI is non-invasive, does not involve ionising radiation, provides a high degree of spatial resolution, and is increasingly available, it may supercede the Wada technique in establishing cerebral dominance for language. Also, other important brain areas - such as those involved in movement - can be identified in a similar way.

Thus, MRI, fMRI, PET, and SPET have significant clinical applications in people with epilepsy because they can identify brain areas containing seizure foci, and those which are essential to higher cognitive (e.g. language) and other (e.g. motor) functions.

## *MRI In General Clinical Practice*

Because it does not use ionising radiation, MRI has radically altered the risk/benefit considerations involved in deciding which patients should undergo brain imaging. People with learning disability have abnormal brain/cognitive function, and this is increasingly amenable to investigation with qualitative and quantitative neuroimaging techniques. In some cases, identification of remediable pathology may lead to improvement in cognitive function, or a decrease in the rate of cognitive decline (for example, in some cases where there is hydocephalus or epilepsy). Therefore, we propose that most patients with learning disability should have at least a baseline structural MRI scan. In some conditions, such as FRAX and Down's Syndrome, where there is known to be structural pathology, there may be uncertainty about the presence of age-related cognitive decline or neuropsychiatric disorder, and such patients should undergo longitudinal MRI studies for comparison. Also, the diagnosis of dementia in people with learning disability is difficult, and decreased hippocampal volume may be a reliable diagnostic marker for Alzheimer's disease in people with Down's Syndrome. Clearly, where patients have localising neurological signs, organic pathology or signs of selective deficits in cognitive function (e.g. memory deficits, or signs of frontal lobe damage), MRI should be performed as it will identify potentially remediable brain abnormalities or allow greater diagnostic certainty. MRI is now an important tool in the investigation of epilepsy, and is essential where this appears to be focal in origin in order to identify the location and type of intracranial abnormalities for future treatment.

Should patients with no sign of underlying progressive brain pathology undergo MRI scanning? In our view, the answer is yes. Such patients are at least, if not more, likely to suffer from intracerebral pathology as the wider population. In the absence of pre-morbid MRI scanning it may not be possible to differentiate the effects of new pathology from those of developmental abnormality.

It is sometimes possible to relate changes in the structure of an individual patient's brain to their behaviour. For example, where there is significant frontal lobe pathology, patients may be socially inappropriate, dis-inhibited, and unmotivated. Such information is also useful in the treatment of behavioural abnormalities. For example, it may be inappropriate to design a treatment programme based upon a particular neuopsychological function (e.g. memory) when a patient has hippocampal and memory abnormalities. Finally, it is often helpful for those involved in the care of a patient to know as far as possible why the patient behaves in a particular way. For example, families may blame themselves for unacceptable aspects of a patient's behaviour, and demonstration of organic pathology may negate this, avoiding recrimination of self or others. Also, correct attribution of a patient's difficulties to specific brain abnormality may enable rehabilitative effort to be concentrated on the patient's strengths rather than weaknesses.

There are infrequent circumstances in which the cost/benefit analysis tilts against scanning. These include issues relating to the provision of informed consent, the need for sedation and any distress that may be caused by the procedure per se.

Finally, brain scanning is a medical procedure, and as such it reinforces the medical model. However, detection and treatment of intracerebral pathology with MRI may decrease morbidity and mortality - particularly in people with a learning disability. Brain scanning with MRI should become part of the routine investigation of pathology in patients with learning disability. Adequate assessment is a patient's right.

## References

Barkowich, A.J., Kjos, B.O., Jackson, D.E. & Norman, D. (1998). Normal maturation of the neonatal and infant brain: MR imaging at 1.5T. *Neuroradiology, 166*, 173-180.

Berardi, A., Haxby, J.V., Grady, C.L & Rapoport S.I. (1990). Memory performance in healthy young and old subjects correlates with resting state brain glucose utilization in the parietal lobe. *Journal of Nuclear Medicine,* 31, 879.

Bruhn, H., Stoppe, G., Merboldt, K.D. et al. (1992). Cereberal metabolic alterations in normal ageing and Altzheimer's demnetia dected by proton MRS. In: Book of Abstracts. Berkeley, California: Society of Magnetic Resonance in Medicine, 752.

Buchsbaum, M.S., Siegel, B.V., Wu, J.C. et al. (1992). Brief report: attention performance in autism and regional brain metabolic rate assessed by positon emission tomography. Journal of Autism and Developmental Disabilities, 22.

Burns, L.H., Pakzaban, P., Deacon, T.W. et al. (1995). Selective putaminal excitotoxic lesions in non-human primates model the movement disorder of Huntington disease. *Neuroscience*, 64, 1007-17.

Chiron, C., Raynaud, C., Maziere, B. et al. (1992). Changes in regional cerebral blood flow during brain maturation in children and adolescents. Journal of Nuclear Medicine, 33, 696-703.

Christophe, C., Muller, M.F., Baleriaux, D. et al. (1990). Mapping of normal brain maturation in infants on phase-sensitive inversion-recovery images. *Neuroradiology*, 3, 173-178.

Chugani, H.T., Phelps, M.E. & Mazziota, J.C. (1987). Positron emission tomography study of human brain functional development. *Annuals of Neurology*, 22, 487-497.

Clark, C., Klonoff, H. & Hayden, M. (1990) Regional cerebral glucose metabolism in Turner Syndrome. *Canadian Journal of Neurological Science,* 17, 140-144.

Coffey, C.E., Wilkinson, W.E., Parashos, I.A. et al. (1992). Quantitative cerebral anatomy of the aging human brain: A cross-sectional study using magnetic resonance imaging. *Neurology,* 42, 527-536.

Courchesne, E., Press, G. & Yeung-Courchesne, R. (1993). Parietal lobe abnormalities detected with MR in patients with infantile autism. *American Journal of Roentgenology,* 160, 387-393.

Courchesne, E., Yeung-Courchesene, R., Press, G. et al. (1988). Hypoplasia of cerebellar vermal lobules V1 and V11 in autism. *New England Journal of Medicine,* 318, 1349-1354.

Cowell, P.E., Turetsky, B.I., Gur, R.C. et al (1994). Sex Differences in Aging of the Human Frontal and Temporal lobes. *Journal of Neuroscience*, 14, 4748-4756.

Curfs, L.M.G., Schreppers-Tijdink, A., Wiegers, A. et al. (1990). The 49 XXXXY syndrome: clinical and psychological findings in five patients. *Journal of Mental Deficiency Research*, 34, 277-282.

de Volder, A., Bol, A., Michel, C. et al. (1987). Brain glucose metabolism in children with the autistic syndrome: positron tomography analysis. *Brain Development*, 9, 581-587.

Debakan, A.S. & Sadowsky, D. (1978). Changes in brain weights during the span of human life: relation of brain weights to body heights and body weights. *Annuals of Neurology*, 4, 345-356.

DeCarli,C.D., Murphy, D.G.M., Gillette, J.A, et al. (1994). Lack of age-related differences in temporal lobe volume of very healthy adults. *American Journal of Neuroradiology*, 15, 689-696.

DeLeo, J.M., Schwartz, M., Creasey, H. et al. (1985). Computer-assisted categorization of brain computerised tomography pixels into cerebrospinal fluid, white matter, and gray matter. *Computerised Biomedical Research*, 18, 79-88.

Egaas, B., Courchesne, E. & Saitoh, O. (1995). Reduced size of corpus callosum in autism. *Archives of Neurology*, 52: 794-801.

Gafney, G.R., Tsai, L.Y., Kuperman, S. et al. (1987). Cerebellar structure in autism. *American Journal of Diseases in Children*, 141, 1330-1332.

Gillberg, I.C., Bjure, J., Uvebrant, P. et al. (1993). SPECT (single photon computed tomography) in 31 children and adolescents with autism and autistic-like conditions. *Child and Adolescent Psychiatry*, 1993, 50-59.

Grady,C.L., McIntosh, A.R., Horwitz, B. et al. (1995). Age-related reductions in human recognition memory due to impaired encoding. *Science,* 269, 218-221.

Harris, G.J., Pearlson, G.D., Peyser, C.E. et al. (1992). Putamen volume reduction on magnetic resonance imaging exceeds caudate changes in mild Huntington's Disease. *Annals of Neurology*, 31, 69-75.

Hashimoto, T., Tayama, M., Miyazaki, M. et al. (1993) Brainstem and cerebellar vermis involvement in autisitc children. *Journal of Child Neurology* , 149-153.

Haxby, J.V. (1989). Neuropsychological evaluation of adults with Down syndrome: patterns of selective impairment in nondemented old adults. *Journal of Mental Deficiency Research,* 33, 193-210.

Horwitz, B., Duara, R. & Rapoport, S.I. (1986). Age differences in intercorrelations between regional cerebral metabolic rates for glucose. *Annuals of Neurology* , 19, 60-67.

Horwitz, B., Rumsey, J.M,, Grady, C.L. & Rapoport, S.I. (1988). The cerebral metabolic lancscape in autism: intercorrelations of regional glucose utilsation. *Archives of Neurology*, 45, 749-755.

Kaye, J.A., DeCarli, C.D., Luxenberg, J.S. & Rapoport, S.I. (1992). The significance of age-related enlargement of the cerebral ventricles in healthy men and women measured by quantitative computed x-ray tomography. *Journal of the American Geriatric Society*, 40, 225-231.

Kemper MB, Hagerman RJ, Ahmad RS, et al (1986). Cognitive profiles and the spectrum of clinical manifestations in heterozygous fragile-X-females. *American Journal of Medical Genetics*, 23, 139-156.

Kemper MB, Hagerman RJ, Altshul-Stark D. (1988). Cognitive profiles of boys with the fragile-X syndrome. *American Journal of Human Genetics*, 30, 191-200.

Kesslak JP, Nagata BS, Lott MD, Nalcoiglu O. (1994). Magnetic resonance imaging analysis of brain age-related changes in the brains of individuals with Down's syndrome. *Neurology*, 44, 1039-1045.

Lotspeich, L. J. & Ciaranello, R. D. (1993). The neurobiology and genetics of infantile autism. *International Review of Neurobiology*, 35, 87-129.

Meyerhoff, D.J., MacKay, S., Constans, J.M. et al. (1992). Axonal injury and membrane alterations in Altzheimer's disease suggested by in vivo proton magnetic resonance spectroscopy imaging. Annuals of Neurology, 36, 40-47.

Miller, B.L., Mouts, R.A., Shonk, T. et al. (1993). N-Astyl Aspartate is decreased by 11% in mild to modertate Altzheimer's disease. *Radiology*, 187, 433-447.

Murakami, J., Courchesne, E, Press, G. et al. (1989). Reduced cerebellar hemisphere size and its relationship to vermal hypoplasia in autism. *Archives of Neurology*, 46, 689-694.

Murata, T., Yoshino, Y., Omori, M. et al. (1993). In vivo proton magnetic resonance spectroscopy study on premature agin gin adult Down's syndrome. *Biological Psychiatry*, 34, 290-297.

Murphy, D.G.M., DeCarli, C.D., Daly, E. et al. (1993). X chromosome effects on female brain:  a magnetic resonance imaging study of Turner's Syndrome. *Lancet,* 342, 1197-1200.

Murphy, D.G.M., DeCarli, C.D., Schapiro, M.B. et al. (1992). Age related differences in volumes of subcortical nuclei, brain matter, and cerebrospinal fluid in healthy men as measured with MRI. *Archives of Neurology,* 49, 839-849.

Murphy, D.G.M., McIntosh, A.R., Daly, E. et al. (1996). Sex differences in human brain morphometry and metabolism: an in vivo quantitative MRI and PET study on the effect of aging. *Archives of General Psychiatry,* 53, 585-594.

Murphy, D.G.M., Mentis, M.J., Pietsini, P. et al. (1997). A PET study of Turner's Syndrome: effects of sex steroids and the X chromosome on brain. *Biological Psychiatry,* 41, 285-298.

Murphy, D.G.M., Mentis, M.J., Grady, C. et al. (1996). Effect of X chromosome triplet repeats on brain glucose metabolism: a PET study of fragile X syndrome premutation carriers. *American Journal of Psychiatry* (submitted).

Pearlson, G.D., Warren, A.C., Starkstein, S.E. et al. (1990). Brain atrophy in 18 patients with Down syndrome: a computed tomographic study. *American Journal of Nuclear Medicine,* 11, 811-816.

Pennington, B., Puck, M. & Robinson, A. (1980). Language and cognitive development of 47 XXX females followed since birth. *Behavioural Genetics,* 10, 31-41.

Reiss, A.L., Abrams, M.T., Greenlaw, R. et al. (1995). Neurodevelopmental effects of the FMR-1 full mutation in humans. *Nature Medicine,* 1: 159-167.

Reiss, A.L., Lee, J. & Freund, L. (1994). Neuroanatomy of fragile X syndrome: the temporal lobe. *Neurology,* 44, 1317-1324.

Rhoades, F.A. (1982). X-linked mental retardation and fragile X or marker X syndrome. *Pediatrics,* 69, 668-669.

Schapiro, M.B., Murphy, D.G.M., Hagerman, R.J. et al. (1995). Adult fragile X syndrome: Neuropsychology, brain anatomy, and metabolism. American Journal of Medical Genetics (Neuropsychiatric Genetics) 60, 480-493.

Sears, L.L., Finn, P.R. & Steinmetz, J.E. (1994). Abnormal classical eye-blink conditioning in autism. *Journal of Autism and Developmental Disorders,* 24, 737-751.

Sedvall, G., Karlsson, P., Lundin, A. et al. (1994). Dopamine D1 receptor number--a sensitive PET marker for early brain degeneration in Huntington's disease. Eur Archives of Psychiatry (Clinical Neuroscience), 243, 249-55.

Shapiro, M.B., Luxenberg, J., Kaye, J. et al. (1989). Serial quantitative CT analysis of brain morphometrics in adult Down Syndrome at different ages. *Neurology,* 39, 1349-1353.

Shetty, U.H., Shapiro, M.B., Holloway, H.W & Rapoport, S.L. (1995). Polyol profiles in Down Syndrome myo-inositol, specifically is elevated in the cerebrospinal fluid. *Journal of Clinical Investigations*, 95, 542-546.

Shonk, T., & Ross, B. (1994). Abstract 2nd Annual Meeting SMR 1994; 600.

Starkstein, S.E., Brandt, J., Folstein, S. et al. (1988). Neuropsychological and neuroradiological correlates in Huntington's disease. *Journal of Neurology and Neurosurgical Psychiatry*, 51, 1259-63.

Takeda, S. & Matsuzawa, T. (1985). Age-related brain atrophy: A study with computed tomography. *Journal of Gerentology*, 40, 159-163.

Veenema, H., Geraedts, J.P.M., Beverstock, G,C, et al. (1987). The fragile-X-syndrome in a large family. Cytogenic and clinical investigations. *Medical Genetics*, 24, 23-31.

Weeks, R.A., Piccini, P., Harding, A.E. et al. (1996). Striatal D1 and D2 dopamine receptor loss in asymptomatic mutation carriers of Huntington's disease. *Annuals of Neurology*, 40, 49-54.

Zilbovicius, M., Garreau, B., Garreau, B. et al. (1995). Delayed maturation of the frontal cortex in childhood autism. *American Journal of Psychiatry* 1995; 152: 248-252.

Zilbovicius M, Garreau B, Tzourio N, et al. (1992). Regional cerebral blood flow in childhood autism: a SPECT study. *American Journal of Psychiatry*, 149, 924-930.

**Dene Robertson** is a clinical lecturer at the Institute of Psychiatry and uses structural and functional imaging techniques to examine brain development and ageing in health and disease. His clinical interests include the assessment and treatment of neuropsychiatric disorder and challenging behaviour in people with a learning disability.

**Declan Murphy** is a senior lecturer at the Institute of Psychiatry; consultant psychiatrist at the Maudsley and Bethlehem Royal Hospitals, and clinical director of the Maudsley Centre for Behaviour Disorders. He has published widely in the fields of neuroimaging, learning disability and brain development.

**Contact Address**
    Department of Psychological Medicine,
    Institute of Psychiatry,
    De Crespigny Park,
    Denmark Hill, London SE 5 8AF